HEALTH SCIENCES LITERATURE REVIEW MADE EASY

THE MATRIX METHOD

JUDITH GARRARD, PhD

PROFESSOR
DIVISION OF HEALTH SERVICES RESEARCH AND POLICY
SCHOOL OF PUBLIC HEALTH
UNIVERSITY OF MINNESOTA
MINNEAPOLIS, MINNESOTA

JONES AND BARTLETT PUBLISHERS
Sudbury, Massachusetts
BOSTON   TORONTO   LONDON   SINGAPORE

World Headquarters
Jones and Bartlett
Publishers
40 Tall Pine Drive
Sudbury, MA 01776
978-443-5000
info@jbpub.com
www.jbpub.com

Jones and Bartlett
Publishers Canada
2406 Nikanna Road
Mississauga, ON L5C
2W6
CANADA

Jones and Bartlett
Publishers
International
Barb House, Barb
Mews
London W6 7PA
UK

Production Credits
Acquisitions Editor: Penny M. Glynn
Production Manager: Amy Rose
Associate Production Editor: Karen C. Ferreira
Editorial Assistant: Amy Sibley
Marketing Manager: Ed McKenna
Cover Designer: Bret Kerr
Cover Photographer: Philip Regan
Manufacturing and Inventory Coordinator: Amy Bacus
Printing and Binding: PA Hutchison
Cover Printing: PA Hutchison

Library of Congress Cataloging-in-Publication Data not available at time
of printing.

Printed in the United States of America
08 07 06 05 04   10 9 8 7 6 5 4 3 2 1

*This book is dedicated to
the grown-up children in my family
who are all such a joy:
Zandy, Heidi, Libby, and Molly, too.*

Table of Contents

Preface

HOW IT BEGAN

For years, as I struggled to meet one grant deadline after another, it became increasingly difficult to keep track of the literature I had reviewed. What I needed was a system that would help me organize my thoughts, as well as the results of my search of the relevant studies. I knew *what* to review and how to assemble all the necessary documents—reprints, photocopies of journal articles, and other materials. What I really needed was a strategy that would make it possible to systematically compare studies on specific topics, to remember exactly which article documented a particular fact (although I knew the article existed), or to quickly and efficiently put my hands on those articles.

What I needed was what I came to call the Matrix Method. Over several years, as I began to develop and use this valuable tool, I discovered that something else was missing: I needed a better filing system. Gradually, I created the Matrix Indexing System. Both methods have given me, my colleagues, and my students tools that make it easier to review and keep track of the scientific literature.

I began to tell students in my graduate courses on research methods and program evaluation about the Matrix Method and the Matrix Indexing System. At first, this consisted of a few comments at the end of a lecture on how to review the literature. Later, I showed them some concrete examples, such as my Lit Review Books, to illustrate the method. These brief sessions grew longer, until I inevitably ran out of class time before I could tell them all they wanted to know. Eventually, these class notes were no longer sufficient. What follows is a full description of the Method and the Indexing System in one small book.

WHO IS THIS BOOK FOR?

This book is intended for people like my graduate students and colleagues, who come from a variety of backgrounds in the health sciences: nurses, physicians, dentists, pharmacists, and graduate students in various public health disciplines, including epidemiology, health services research, environmental health, public health nursing, health education, public health administration, and health care management. Occasionally I have had graduate students from disciplines outside of the health sciences—sociology, psychology, anthropology, social work, demography, and geography—and they, too, have found the Matrix Method useful.

While this book will prove a useful tool to people of many different levels of knowledge and understanding about research methods, those who perhaps will find it most useful are the students who took my beginning research methods course in the School of Public Health. These are people of varied background and preparation, who have had a wide range of work experiences, with a majority in health related fields.

Students are not the only ones who can use such a book. Clinicians in the health professions—physicians, nurses, dentists, pharmacists—are being urged by leaders in their fields to rely more on the research literature for making clinical decisions, and they, too, need a system for conducting and organizing such reviews. Others who will have use for this book are those in academic settings; the health care industry, including managed care organizations, hospitals, and nursing homes; the pharmaceutical industry; the nonprofit sector; county and state health departments; and public health programs. All of these people have a need to master the research literature in their own fields. This book can serve as a guide through that process as well as provide a method for organizing both thinking and source materials about the scientific literature.

Whether for students, clinicians, researchers, policy analysts, or other information professionals, the Matrix Method is a useful tool. This book goes beyond other books that describe how to analyze a scientific study, or interpret the literature,[1] or integrate research studies using techniques such as meta-analysis.[2] Instead, the Matrix Method provides a way to review and organize the literature. It is a system for bringing order out of the chaos of too much information spread across too many sources in too many places.

FEEDBACK, PLEASE

No matter how many students or colleagues there are to discuss concepts or how exciting it is to debate different points, writing is essentially a singular activity. Rarely is there the opportunity to hear from the people who actually use the finished product. Knowing how much the book has benefited from these interactions as it was being written, I welcome comments about these results. Let me know which parts of the Matrix Method and the Matrix Indexing System worked or didn't work and tell me what else is needed. It has been a pleasure to write this book. I hope you find it useful.

Judith Garrard, PhD
University of Minnesota
Minneapolis, Minnesota
jgarrard@tc.umn.edu

REFERENCES

1. Gehlbach SH. Interpreting the Medical Literature. 3rd ed. NY: McGraw-Hill; 1993.
2. Cooper HM. Integrating Research: A Guide for Literature Reviews. Newbury Park, CA: Sage Publications; 1989.

Acknowledgments

I am indebted to many colleagues, students, and friends who contributed their time, expertise, and support in the writing and producing of this book. Let me begin by thanking the reference librarians and staff of the University of Minnesota Biomedical Library: Julie Kelly, Delbert Reed, Mary G. Mueller, Dawn Littleton, Janet Arth, M. Kathryn Robbins, and Gail Weinberg. Students and colleagues at the University of Minnesota were also very helpful: Michele Cleary, Neil Jordan, Margaret Artz, Mary E. S. Indritz, Melinda Voss, Joan Langlois, Carla Kahle, Tim Lindholm, Helen Nelson, Sarah Trachet, Marsha Finklestein, Kathleen Call, Elizabeth Gustin, Toni Toledo, Joan Bushman, Pat Bland, Cynthia Gross, Margaret Bull, Bernie Feldman, Sara De Hart, Joan Garfield, Robert Kane, and Richard A. Krueger. I am especially indebted to Susan Harms for her support and discussions about the ideas in this book. Karen Virnig has been a major source of support. Students, faculty, and friends from outside of the University of Minnesota were also very helpful: Nancy Leland, Carol Skay, Terry Foley, Jane Pederson, Andrew Langlois, Jenny Staben, and my undergraduate expert, Amy Boedicker. Finally, I am grateful to my husband, Bill Garrard, for his encouragement and support.

The author and publisher are grateful for permission to reprint copyrighted materials from each of the following:

- Netscape and the Netsite logo
- OVID
- Niles Software, Inc. for references to EndNote®
- Institute for Scientific Information for references to Current Contents®
- The American Public Health Association for reference to articles in the *American Journal of Public Health*
- The Gerontological Society of America for reference to an article in *The Gerontologist*
- Cochrane Collaboration

Fundamentals of a Literature Review

Introduction

The Matrix Method is a versatile strategy for reviewing the literature. The background and philosophy of a literature review and an introduction to the Matrix Method are described in the following sections in this chapter:

- ☑ Review of the Literature
- ☑ Beyond Index Cards
- ☑ To Own the Literature
- ☑ Research Synthesis: Historical Perspective
- ☑ The Matrix Method: Definition and Overview
- ☑ Review Matrix: A Versatile Tool
- ☑ Overview of Chapters and Appendix
- ☑ References to Web Sites
- ☑ Caroline's Quest: Understanding the Process

REVIEW OF THE LITERATURE

The purpose of this book is to describe the Matrix Method and the Matrix Indexing System. The Matrix Method is a strategy for reviewing the literature, especially the scientific literature. A review of the literature consists of reading, analyzing, and summarizing scholarly materials about a specific topic. When the review is of scientific literature, the focus is on the hypotheses, scientific methods, results, strengths and weaknesses of the study, and the authors' interpretations and conclusions. A review of the scientific literature is fundamental to understanding the accumulated knowledge about the topic being reviewed. The Matrix Indexing System helps the user to create and maintain a reprint file.

The term *scientific literature* refers to theoretical and research publications in scientific journals, reference books, textbooks, government reports, policy statements, and other materials about the theory, practice, and results of scientific inquiry. These materials and publications are produced by individuals or groups in universities, foundations, government research laboratories, and other nonprofit or for-profit organizations. Currently, the most common type of publication used in a review of up-to-date scientific literature is a research paper in a scientific journal, such as the *Journal of the American Medical Association* or the *American Journal of Epidemiology*.

Reviews of the literature are the foundation for developing grant proposals, research papers, summary articles, books, policy and regulatory statements, and consumer materials. Given the vast number of scientific publications produced over the past several decades, information retrieval and analysis in the form of a critical review of the literature has become more crucial than ever.

BEYOND INDEX CARDS

In the past, most students conducted their first review of the literature in high school or college when they learned how to do library research. Usually their efforts concentrated on where to gather information and how to use the library. With the explosion in use of computers over the past 25 years, students now learn about electronic information retrieval at the primary school level.

Using computers to retrieve information is not the only new development, however. The amount of information to be examined and critiqued has increased exponentially over the past 50 years. This decade alone has witnessed tremendous advancements in scientific knowledge, a dramatic increase in the number of scientific journals, and a bewildering array of new forms of communication. Books and scientific journals are no longer the only venue for scholarly literature. Information is available on the Internet, in worldwide meetings of professional societies, and in correspondence by e-mail. How, where, when, and whether or not to obtain such information constitute a present-day dilemma for anyone who reviews the literature. The art of conducting such a review is an entirely separate matter.

Formal instruction in how to systematically organize and carry out a review of the literature is rarely offered in educational programs at any level, including graduate school. In the past, American students were advised to use index cards to record the most salient points of the material being reviewed. In recent years, many students have begun to keep their notes on a computer. Despite such technological advances, how to avoid getting lost in the details between generating a computer list of research articles, accumulating a stack of index cards or notes on a word processor, and writing the final synthesis is still something of a mystery to many people.

One way of mastering this process is to realize that a review of any body of literature is really four tasks in one. Reviewers have to

- make decisions about which documents to review,
- read and understand what the authors present,
- evaluate the ideas, research methods, and results of each publication, and
- write a synthesis that includes both the content and a critical analysis of these materials.

Given the complexity of each one of these tasks, it is easy to become overwhelmed in the process. A strategy is needed to organize the books and papers selected in the search and retrieval process; structure the information in order to understand the progression of ideas by different authors across documents and over time; and use that structure to develop a critique and write a synthesis of the results of such a review. The Matrix Method provides such a strategy.

TO OWN THE LITERATURE

There is something else that can result from a thorough and comprehensive review of the literature that may be even more valuable than a written synthesis: ownership of the literature. To "own the literature," you must *know* it—know the major ideas, what has been researched, the names of the authors and where they are located, who collaborated with whom, what databases they did (or did not) use, the strengths and weaknesses of the studies, what has been studied ad infinitum, and what is missing.

To own the literature is to be so familiar with what has been written by previous researchers that you know clearly how this area of research has progressed over time and across ideas. Without a thorough and comprehensive review of the literature, you are at the mercy of every critic and reviewer who *is* aware of what is known, how it evolved, and what has yet to be examined.

Unfortunately, such ownership cannot be acquired easily: you have to complete the whole process of a literature review, from the initial search to the final written synthesis, before you can take possession of the literature on a subject. Ownership is rarely mentioned when people describe the literature in a paper or presentation, but it exists, and experienced reviewers achieve such ownership whether or not they realize it.

When you own the literature, you are in a better position to know what is missing in a stream of research, you can defend your ideas, and you can anticipate what other scientists and researchers will say or do. Ownership is the mastery of how a specific body of knowledge evolved, what it currently comprises, and what has yet to be studied.

Acquiring ownership of a literature demands more than summarizing the studies or documents you review. A summary merely describes. Your task is to read and analyze each document until you can picture what the authors did in a study or the logical process they went through in making a point. Then you must go back and critically analyze what was right and wrong each step of the way. To own the literature is to dissect each part and decide whether or not you agree with what the authors did or said. In other words, you must become engaged with the content, argue with the authors, and conclude for yourself if this paper or study made sense from a scientific or scholarly standpoint. You must understand how the field has evolved: the progression of ideas over time and across different authors. To own the literature you must learn about the conceptual models that served as the foundation for the research. Deduce what hypotheses were really being tested, who initiated the ideas, and who did the first research study. The Matrix Method will help you acquire ownership of the literature, but it is only a guide. The most important component is your active involvement with the literature.

RESEARCH SYNTHESIS: HISTORICAL PERSPECTIVE

Overview

Before delving into the details of the Matrix Method, it might be useful to think about the historical context of a review of the literature. A literature review is part of the larger endeavor of research synthesis that is the analysis, interpretation, and use of scientific inquiry. Although the term *research synthesis* can be applied to all kinds of knowledge, this discussion will be limited to some examples of how the synthesis of health sciences research literature has evolved. The practices and tools used today for reviewing the health sciences literature can be traced back to 1879 with the publishing of *Index*

Medicus, a medical bibliography that included a subject and author index to articles published in medical journals.[1] Today's most useful tools, however, are relatively recent innovations. An historical awareness of how the research literature has grown and when some of these tools were introduced will help put these developments into perspective.

Since the mid-1940s, the number of scientific publications has increased dramatically. What spurred this increase is complicated and best left to social and medical historians to explain, but certainly a major factor has been a concomitant rise in the amount of funding for research by the National Institutes of Health. These growth rates are shown in Figure 1-1. In this example, publications are those defined by the *Science Citation Index* as original substantive articles, editorial materials, letters, reports of meetings, correction notes, and reviews for the period from 1945 to 1996.[2,3] The NIH dollars are those allocated for research grants.[4]

Some critics suggest that there is no evidence of an increase in the rate of scientific publications over time, citing two reasons for this rationale: (1) the quantity of scientific publications has increased but not the quality[5] and (2) the rate of publications per health scientist has remained the same, but the number of health scientists has increased.[6] Neither argument addresses the fact that an individual health scientist today must cope with an increase in the absolute number of journals and publications that have to be considered when reviewing the literature.

In examining the growth rates in Figure 1-1, the increase in NIH grant dollars may not be as steep as indicated because the figures are actual dollars spent for each 5-year period, unadjusted for inflation. The real rate of growth may be flatter or dip more in some years than others, once inflation has been taken into account. But for the sake of argument, consider the two rates of growth at their face value and assume an upward trajectory for both.

What is important is the juxtaposition of the growth in the number of publications, the amount of research funding, and developments in resources for creating a synthesis of the re-

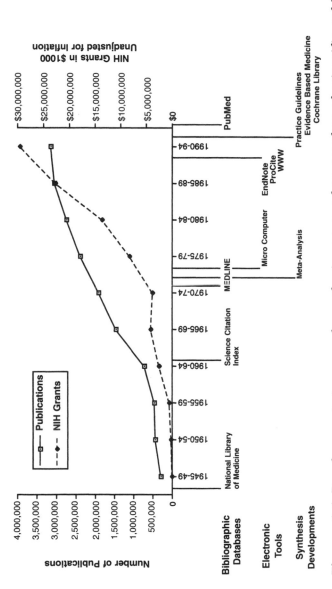

Figure 1-1 Developments in research synthesis compared to number of scientific publications and funding for research grants from the National Institutes of Health (NIH). *Source:* Data about publications from Science Citation Index 1945–1954 Cumulative Comparative Statistical Summary, in *SCI Science Citation Index Ten Year Cumulation 1945–1954: Guide and Lists of Source Publications*, pp. 18–19, © 1988, Institute for Scientific Information; and Comparative Statistical Summary 1955–1996, in *SCI Science Citation Index 1996 Annual Guide and Lists of Source Publications*, pp. 57–63, © 1997, Institute for Scientific Information. Data about NIH research funds from NIH Almanac 1997, in Branch EO, Publication No. 97-5, 1997, National Institutes of Health.

search literature. Examples of these developments over the past 50 years can be assigned to three categories: (1) the establishment of bibliographic databases, (2) the creation of electronic tools for manipulating information, and (3) the emergence of synthesis applications.

Bibliographic Databases

Bibliographic databases include information in print and electronic form. The first major development in this category for the health sciences was the creation of the National Library of Medicine (NLM) under the aegis of the Public Health Service of the Department of Health, Education, and Welfare. The NLM evolved from the Library of the Army Surgeon General's Office, which was established in 1836.[1] With major funding from Congress in 1942, the NLM established a national collection of scientific books, papers, and reports located in Washington, DC. Accessing this information electronically was difficult for scientists in other parts of the country, one that was only partially solved in 1961 with the creation of the *Science Citation Index*, and later its sister application, the *Social Science Citation Index* by Eugene Garfield. These indexes are owned and published by the Institute for Scientific Information®. Their Internet address is: http://www.isinet.com/.

In 1971, MEDLINE®, an electronic database of the scientific literature in medical and other health related journals and publications, was launched by the NLM and became one of the premier tools for the health sciences researcher. Initially, access to MEDLINE was brokered by reference librarians, which made frequent or spontaneous use awkward in the daily life of most scientists. Such use could also be expensive; a charge per reference had a chilling effect on the financially strapped graduate student or unfunded assistant professor—the very users who most needed such access.

The rules for searching MEDLINE were also complicated. Reference librarians had to undergo specialized training in order to master the intricacies of the search, and not all research libraries had specialized personnel. Nonetheless, the availability of an electronic database that could be searched to locate specific studies was a major advantage for the health scientist engaged in some aspect of research synthesis.

Gradually, an infrastructure for an electronic bibliographic database became more refined, with standardized key words and more easily understood rules for creating a search strategy. Although the scientist intent on using the electronic version of MEDLINE was still bound to one of the research libraries, and bound even more tightly to the services of a knowledgeable librarian, this ability to access the research literature was a major advantage. The number of research publications had already begun an upswing by this point in time. This is reflected in the rate of growth shown in Figure 1-1 for the period after MEDLINE became available, although cause and effect have not been clearly established between the development and the rate.

The period since MEDLINE's inception has seen the creation of a myriad of other bibliographic databases, such as Psyc INFO, International Pharmaceutical Abstracts, and CINAHL. The final example in Figure 1-1 of a development in this category of bibliographic databases is PubMed, which was launched in 1997 and provides worldwide access to MEDLINE on the Internet. Anyone, scientist or layperson, now has access to the MEDLINE database of over 9 million references just by signing onto its website at www.ncbi.nlm.nih.gov/ PubMed/. Not only is PubMed free, the use of MEDLINE is no longer bounded geographically to a library or restricted by the availability of a qualified librarian. All that is needed is a computer and access to the Internet.

Electronic Tools

Only a few examples of developments in the second category, that of electronic tools, will be described, beginning with the microcomputer. Without a doubt, the introduction in the mid-1970s of a reasonably priced personal computer represents a seminal event in any historical description of the late twentieth century. For the reviewer of the literature, the availability of a personal computer vastly improved the quality of academic life. Word processing software, together with information in bibliographic databases, made the tasks of searching and abstracting the scientific literature far more efficient.

There continued to be other problems, however, one of which was the lack of a standardized format for citations and references to articles in scientific journals or books. If a health scientist had to switch from one formatting system to another in the preparation of a paper or report, he or she was forced to go back through the entire document and make the changes one by one. Although there is still no single, universal format, another kind of solution was developed. In the late 1980s, two reference management software packages were produced that made changes from one formatting system to another automatically, thus providing some relief for the time-strapped researcher. Both software products were created by academicians. EndNote® was introduced in 1988 and ProCite® in 1989. Not only do these two software packages satisfy their original intent of allowing the user to switch from one reference formatting system to another, but they now have additional features such as the creation of a reference library on the user's own computer, a search and sort capability, a seamless download of a reference and its abstract from electronic bibliographic databases to desktop computers, and the flexibility of user-defined information for each reference.

The impact of reference management software packages does not equal that of the personal computer in a list of important developments in the history of research synthesis or information management. Nevertheless, these software products are good solid tools for everyday use and are like a set of well-honed kitchen utensils compared to the discovery of fire: the latter is necessary, but once that is available, the former makes the job easier.

Like the personal computer, another advance comparable to the "discovery of fire" was the establishment of the World Wide Web in 1989. With the Web, individual researchers have the capability of free and unlimited worldwide access to information, not only between each other, but also to banks of information such as the electronic bibliographic databases and other scientific forums that have rapidly proliferated. The use of these electronic tools in combination with bibliographic databases, together with an increase in the absolute number of scientific publications and NIH grant dollars, contributed to developments in the third category of development—that of synthesis applications.

Synthesis Applications

It is easy to imagine that if the same rate of growth in scientific publications had been seen in the financial market, investors would have been ecstatic with joy. There was more research, better science, and an exponential growth in new information, but the scientific community pondered how to make use of it. How could this growing reservoir of scientific knowledge be managed and used for the betterment of humankind, or at the least, for individual patients? Three developments in the late 1990s illustrate a response to these questions: practice guidelines, evidence-based medicine, and the Cochrane reviews of clinical trials. These developments are shown at the far right of the timeline in Figure 1-1. Prior to their appearance, however, a new methodological technique, meta-analysis, was proposed in the mid-1970s, just before personal computers and the Web became available.

Meta-Analysis. A professor of education, Gene Glass, was one of the first to outline a way of statistically summarizing the results of multiple studies on the same topic. His initial paper was published in 1976.[7] Health scientists quickly saw the advantage of this technique and began to apply it to biomedical research studies. The use of this and other techniques contributed to the subsequent development of prime examples of synthesis applications in the 1990s:

- Clinical practice guidelines generated largely by the Americans

- Evidence-based medicine created almost single-handedly by the Canadians
- Reviews by the worldwide Cochrane Collaboration led by the British

All of these resulted from national and international collaborations, made possible by local, national, and international funding. These developments depend on the resources of bibliographic databases, electronic tools, and an intense commitment to making use of available research findings to improve the health care of the individual and the public.

Clinical Practice Guidelines. Practice guidelines were developed with the intention of providing practitioners, such as physicians, nurses, and allied health professionals, with sound strategies based on the scientific literature for delivering the best possible health care. A formal definition of a clinical practice guideline was provided by the Institute of Medicine in 1992.

In 1993, the first Practice Guideline was commissioned and funded by the Agency for Health Care Policy and Research (AHCPR), a federal granting agency created by Congress in 1989. Over the following 5 years, AHCPR commissioned Practice Guidelines on 19 topics that were published between 1992 and 1998. Examples of topics include acute pain management, depression in primary care, HIV infection, otitis media with effusion in children, and post-stroke rehabilitation.

In conjunction with the American Association of Health Plans and the American Medical Association, AHCPR developed the National Guideline Clearinghouse web site, http://www.guideline.gov/, dedicated to enhancing access to the guidelines in 1998. (An alternative web site for a listing of AHCPR guidelines is: http://text.nlm.nih.gov/ftrs/pick?/collect =ahcpr&dbName=0&cc=1&t=898717327/.) Currently, AHCPR has redefined its role as that of facilitator to other organizations such as specialty societies or managed care organizations or local groups of clinicians in their development of future practice guidelines.

Evidence-Based Medicine. The basic concepts of evidence-based medicine were conceived by a group of academicians at

McMaster University in Hamilton, Ontario, led by Professor G. H. Guyatt. Their web site is: http://hiru.mcmaster.ca/. The medical school at McMaster has long been known for its innovativeness in medical education, and these clinician-scholars expanded their audience from a classroom of medical students in southern Canada to health care providers throughout the world.

Guyatt and his colleagues recognized the need for members of the medical community to improve their ability to evaluate and use the scientific literature.[8] An ongoing series of Users' Guides, published in the *Journal of the American Medical Association (JAMA)*, has provided a set of tutorials for clinicians on such diverse topics as how to use articles about diagnosis, prognosis, grading health care recommendations, and applicability of clinical trial results. A list of such articles from 1993 to 1998 is provided in the Appendix.[8-27] A web site that provides a wide array of resources for exploring evidence-based practice can be found at http://www.shef.ac.uk/uni/academic/R-Z/scharr/ir/netting.html/.

The concepts of evidence-based medicine have been adopted by clinicians in other disciplines, including nursing, dentistry, and pharmacy. A term with broader application has begun to emerge, that of evidence-based practice. The relationship between evidence-based practice and clinical practice guidelines has not been fully examined, although, logically, they are closely linked. Clearly, what they have in common is a foundation of scientific literature that has been carefully reviewed and systematically abstracted. At its simplest, evidence-based practice is what a practitioner such as a physician or nurse-clinician does one-on-one with a patient; whereas, practice guidelines provide guidance for best clinical practice.

The Cochrane Collaboration. An example of the most recent development of a synthesis application is that of the Cochrane Library, an electronic library of systematic reviews of the clinical literature created and maintained by the Cochrane Collaboration.

In 1992, a nonprofit organization, the Cochrane Centre, was created in Oxford, England, in response to concerns expressed

20 years earlier by Archie Cochrane, a British epidemiologist.[28] An outgrowth of the Centre was the establishment in 1993 of the Cochrane Collaboration, an international, voluntary, collaborative effort to provide systematic and critical reviews of randomized controlled trials of health care.[29] Participants in the collaboration are organized through collaborative review groups that include researchers, health care professionals, and consumers throughout the world, including experts in the U.S. and Canada.

The ongoing mission of the Cochrane Collaboration is to prepare, maintain, and promote the accessibility of systematic reviews of the effects of health care interventions. Current information about the Cochrane Collaboration can be found at http://www.cochrane.co.uk/.

The Cochrane Collaboration is an example of the international, multidisciplinary nature of the current field of research synthesis. Communication is rapid and easily accessible via the Internet. Information available in the Cochrane Library can be readily obtained by lay audiences. Thus the Cochrane Library has an important role to play in the democratization of health care information. The availability of the Cochrane Library is very recent, dating back to the mid-1990s following the creating of the Cochran Collaboration in 1993. The further development and impact of this resource for health professionals and consumers bear close scrutiny in the future.

This brief history of the emergence of the field of research synthesis in the health sciences has focused exclusively on developments in English language systems, and largely in North America, with some mention of the role of the British. Linguistic and geographic boundaries of science are disappearing daily, however, and the full scope of developments and use of research synthesis cannot be confined to a single language or these few countries.

In the future, the history of research synthesis will need a broader cultural and linguistic perspective in order to provide a complete understanding of the impact of this field on the health of people. The role of the Internet, the importance of multidisciplinary collaboration, and access to scientific knowledge by people who are not health professionals will also be important factors in understanding how research synthesis can have an impact on the health and lives of people throughout the world.

For the present, the surfeit of information in the health sciences literature and the resources that have emerged in recent years to assist in reviewing and synthesizing that information present both a challenge and an opportunity. A systematic way of conducting a literature review incorporating the efficient use of those resources is needed. The Matrix Method offers one such system.

THE MATRIX METHOD: DEFINITION AND OVERVIEW

The Matrix Method is both a structure and a process for systematically reviewing the literature. The structure is provided by a Lit Review Book—a binder such as a 3-ring notebook, that contains all of the notes and documentation accumulated in conducting a review of the literature. The Lit Review Book is divided into 4 major sections, as shown in Exhibit 1-1, consisting of the following:

- **Paper Trail—Keeping Track of Where You've Been.** This is a record of the search process used to identify relevant materials. Examples include notes about the materials examined, key words used to search the electronic bib-

Exhibit 1-1 Structure of the Matrix Method: Four Sections of the Lit Review Book

- Paper Trail—Keeping Track of Where You've Been

- Documents Section—Organizing Documents for Review

- Review Matrix—Abstracting Each Document

- Synthesis—Writing the Review of the Literature

liographic databases in the library, and instructions for electronic searches.

- **Documents Section—Organizing Documents for Review.** This section includes a photocopy of all of the journal articles, book chapters, and other materials gathered for your review of the literature. These are the documents used to create a Review Matrix, which is the third section.
- **Review Matrix—Abstracting Each Document.** This is a sheet of paper (or a spreadsheet on your computer) with columns and rows that you use to abstract selected information about each journal article, book chapter, or other materials included in your review of the literature.
- **Synthesis—Writing the Review of the Literature.** This is the outcome of your use of the Matrix Method, a written synthesis of your critical review of the literature based on the materials you abstracted in the Review Matrix.

The Lit Review Book does not have to be a 3-ring notebook. It might also be a virtual book in the form of a computer file for all but the Documents Section, which contains a photocopy or reprint of the documents you abstract. Even the Documents Section could be stored on a computer once all papers and documents become available in electronic form. Until that time, however, a hard copy of the Documents Section is necessary. Rather than alternate between describing a hard copy, 3-ring notebook and a virtual copy on a computer, this book will describe the hard copy version of the Lit Review Book, which may be converted to the electronic version.

In addition to structure in the form of a Lit Review Book, the Matrix Method also provides a process for how to create and use the materials in each of the 4 sections. That process is described in Chapters 3 through 6. The Matrix Method was specifically designed for reviews of the health sciences literature, but it can be used for reviews of the literature in any field by anyone at any level of expertise, from novice to seasoned reviewer. The key to the versatility of the Matrix Method lies in the use of the Review Matrix, which is described briefly here and is explained in greater detail in Chapter 5.

REVIEW MATRIX: A VERSATILE TOOL

With a Review Matrix you create a structured abstract of all of the documents in your literature review. A Review Matrix is like a spreadsheet—a rectangular arrangement of columns and rows. All that is needed to set up a blank Review Matrix is a pencil and piece of paper to create the blank forms. Large tabulation sheets available in office supply stores are also useful. Alternatively, a blank Review Matrix can be created on a computer using a word processor or a spreadsheet such as Microsoft Excel.

The columns across the top of a Review Matrix are the topics or headings you use to abstract each document or study. The rows down the page are the documents or studies. The point at which each column and row meets is a cell, which is where you write notes about a document. An example of the format for a Review Matrix is shown in Exhibit 1-2, in which there are 4 columns and 2 rows. Each column has a topic, such as author-title-journal or year, and each row consists of a journal article. Thus, the Review Matrix is a place to record notes about each article, paper, study, or document on the basis of a standard set of column topics.

Column topics can range from the very general to the specific. For example, a Review Matrix for Shakespeare's plays might include these column topics: Setting, Characters, Protagonist, Antagonist, and Psychological Theme. Alternatively, if the focus was on the scientific literature, the Matrix would feature other kinds of column topics: Hypothesis, Independent Variable, Dependent Variable, Methodological Design, and Sampling Design.

No matter the level of expertise or area of focus, you are entirely in control of the Review Matrix. You decide which column topics to use and which documents or studies to review. The process you use to make those decisions—which

Exhibit 1-2 Example of the Format of a Review Matrix

Column #1	Column #2	Column #3	Column #4
Example: Author, title, journal	Example: Year	Example: Purpose	Example: Type of Study Design
Row #1 Journal article #1	1995	Drug treatment for epilepsy	Experimental study
Row #2 Journal article #2	1997	Drug treatment for depression	Case-control study

topics, which documents—is described in this book. In the course of making those decisions, abstracting the articles, and writing the synthesis, you begin to take ownership of the literature.

OVERVIEW OF CHAPTERS AND APPENDIX

The creation and use of the Review Matrix and Lit Review Book are described in the remaining chapters. Although the Matrix Method can be applied to the literature on just about any topic, there is an emphasis throughout this book on the health sciences. The 9 chapters in this book are organized into 3 sections:

- Part I. Fundamentals of a Literature Review—Chapters 1 and 2
- Part II. The Matrix Method—Chapters 3 through 6
- Part III. Applications Using the Matrix Method—Chapters 7 through 9

Chapters 2 through 9 are described briefly below, followed by an overview of Appendix A. At the end of each chapter is a section titled *Caroline's Quest*, which includes practical examples of how the concepts can be applied.

Chapter 2, Basic Concepts

This chapter consists of definitions of concepts that are fundamental in any review of the literature, and especially those used in the Matrix Method. Also included in this chapter is a description of the different parts of a typical scientific paper published in most health related journals. If you know where to find specific topics, then you will be in a better position to abstract the study. Chapter 2 also describes the basic elements of a methodological review of the literature. These elements can be used as the sole basis of a review, or more realistically, as a list of possibilities for inclusion, together with the content of the field under review. A list of potential column topics for reviewing the research methodology in the scientific literature is given in the section, Guidelines for a Methodological Review of the Literature.

Chapter 3, Paper Trail: How To Plan and Manage a Search of the Literature

This chapter describes what steps to take in doing a review of the literature, how to develop a key words list, how to locate source materials, how to use the snowballing technique, what to consider in a computer search of established databases such as MEDLINE, Psyc INFO, Science Citation Index, and use of the Internet.

Chapter 4, Documents Section: How To Select and Organize Documents for Review

This chapter includes a description of how to choose documents and organize journal articles and other source materials. The advantages of maintaining a chronologically ordered set of photocopied articles in a 3-ring binder are also discussed.

Chapter 5, Review Matrix: How To Abstract the Research Literature

The Review Matrix is the heart of the Matrix Method. This chapter describes how to set up a Review Matrix, including issues such as choosing topics to abstract, variations in topics, addition of topics later in the process, and a step-by-step guide for constructing the Review Matrix.

Chapter 6, Synthesis: How To Use a Review Matrix To Write a Synthesis

This chapter is a description of how to use the Review Matrix to critically analyze and write a review of the literature, including a discussion of differences between a summary and a synthesis.

Chapter 7, A Library of Lit Review Books

This chapter describes the advantages of maintaining a collection of Lit Review Books for use over time, or by a team of people, or across interrelated topics. Specifics include how to create and expand a library of Lit Review Books.

Chapter 8, The Matrix Indexing System

This chapter describes a system for integrating information from electronic databases and reference libraries created with reference management software and copies of papers in the Documents Section of the Lit Review Book. The advantages of this system are discussed, together with information about how to set up and use such a system.

Chapter 9, Matrix Applications by Health Sciences Professionals

This chapter describes 4 kinds of applications for the experienced health sciences professional. These include the use of the Matrix Method in (1) conducting a research project, from writing a grant proposal to publishing the results; (2) standardizing the review process for a meta-analysis; (3) creating and using clinical practice guidelines; and (4) applying the concepts of evidence-based medicine.

Appendix, Useful Resources for Literature Reviews

This is a handy list of books, journals, and Internet websites that can be useful in searching further for scientific literature that is not available in the standard sources. The Appendix is a potpourri of useful information.

REFERENCES TO WEB SITES

Web site addresses on the Internet are given throughout the remaining chapters and especially in the Appendix. Each address on the Internet, called a Universal Resource Locator (URL), was examined and determined to be accurate and functional at the time this book went to press, but the Internet is a dynamic environment, and URLs can change on an hourly basis. For this reason, neither the author nor the publisher is responsible for the accuracy of the URLs provided in this book.

Caroline's Quest:
Understanding the Process

Just as a picture can be worth a thousand words in explaining a concept, a practical example can be equally valuable in demonstrating a process. With that in mind, each of the 9 chapters in this book will conclude with a description of the experiences of a typical graduate student, Caroline Collins, as she learns about Matrix applications and uses the Matrix Method and the Matrix Indexing System in reviewing the literature for her master's thesis in public health.

Caroline tends to be a bit impatient and will occasionally try to take shortcuts in order to avoid some of the more time-consuming details of the Matrix Method. Fortunately, she meets weekly with her advisor, Professor Dickerson, who gives her advice about using the Matrix applications. Caroline's experiences and Professor Dickerson's explanations illustrate not only the process but also the rationale for why certain steps in the Matrix Method are needed and how the Matrix Indexing System can help her organize her materials.

In medieval times, a quest was a chivalrous enterprise involving an adventurous journey that often required courage or determination. In modern times, a quest is defined as a search or pursuit. Although Caroline does not have to deal with dragons in the library, her review of the literature does require persistence and determination in her pursuit of knowledge, a pursuit that is occasionally adventurous. Thus, in both the modern and the ancient senses of the word, Caroline has embarked upon a quest.

REFERENCES

1. National Library of Medicine. Images from the history of the public health service: Biomedical research. Available at: http://www.nlm.nih.gov/exhibition/phs_history/99.html. Accessed September 24, 1998.

2. Institute for Scientific Information. Science Citation Index 1945–1954 Cumulative Comparative Statistical Summary. In *SCI Science Citation Index Ten Year Cumulation 1945–1954: Guide and Lists of Source Publications*. Philadelphia: Institute for Scientific Information;1988: 18–19.

3. Institute for Scientific Information. Comparative Statistical Summary 1955–1996. In *SCI Science Citation Index 1996 Annual Guide and Lists of Source Publications*. Philadelphia: Institute for Scientific Information; 1997:57–63.

4. National Institutes of Health. NIH Almanac 1997. Washington DC: NIH Publication No 97-5; 1997. (Internet version of the Almanac available at: http://www.nih.gov/welcome/almanac 97/toc.htm/)

5. Garfield E. In truth, the "flood" of scientific literature is only a myth. *The Scientist*. 1991;5:11–25.

6. Huth EJ. The information explosion. *Bull NY Acad Med*. 1989;65: 647–661.

7. Glass G. Primary, secondary, and meta-analysis of research. *Educational Researcher*. 1976;5:3–8.

8. Guyatt GH, Rennie D. Users' Guides to the Medical Literature. *JAMA*. 1993;270:2096–2097.

9. Oxman AD, Sackett DL, Guyatt GH. Users' guides to the medical literature: I. How to get started. *JAMA*. 1993;270:2093–2095.

10. Guyatt GH, Sackett DL, Cook DJ, Evidence-Based Medicine Working Group. Users' guides to the medical literature. II. How to use an article about therapy or prevention. A. Are the results of the study valid? *JAMA*. 1993;270:2598–2601.

11. Guyatt GH, Sackett DL, Cook DJ, Evidence-Based Medicine Working Group. Users' guides to the medical literature. II. How to use an article about therapy or prevention. B. What were the results and will they help me in caring for my patients? *JAMA*. 1994;271:59–63.

12. Jaeschke R, Guyatt G, Sackett DL, Evidence-Based Medicine Working Group. Users' guide to the medical literature. III. How to use an article about a diagnostic test. A. Are the results of the study valid? *JAMA*. 1994;271:389–391.

13. Jaeschke R, Guyatt GH, Sackett DL, Evidence-Based Medicine Working Group. Users' guides to the medical literature. III. How to use an article

about a diagnostic test. B. What are the results and will they help me in caring for my patients? *JAMA*. 1994;271:703–707.

14. Levine M, Walter S, Lee H, Evidence-Based Medicine Working Group. Users' guides to the medical literature. IV. How to use an article about harm. *JAMA*. 1994;271:1615–1619.

15. Laupacis A, Wells G, Richardson WS, Tugwell P, Evidence-Based Medicine Working Group. Users' guides to the medical literature. V. How to use an article about prognosis. *JAMA*. 1994;272:234–237.

16. Oxman AD, Cook DJ, Guyatt GH, Evidence-Based Medicine Working Group. Users' guides to the medical literature. VI. How to use an overview. *JAMA*. 1994;272:1367–1371.

17. Richardson WS, Detsky AS, Evidence-Based Medicine Working Group. Users' guides to the medical literature. VII. How to use a clinical decision analysis. A. Are the results of the study valid? *JAMA*. 1995;273: 1292–1295.

18. Richardson WS, Detsky AS, Evidence-Based Medicine Working Group. Users' guides to the medical literature. VII. How to use a clinical decision analysis. B. What are the results and will they help me in caring for my patients? *JAMA*. 1995;273:1610–1613.

19. Hayward RS, Wilson MC, Tunis SR, Bass EB, Guyatt G, Evidence-Based Medicine Working Group. Users' guides to the medical literature. VIII. How to use clinical practice guidelines. A. Are the recommendations valid? *JAMA*. 1995;274:570–574.

20. Wilson MC, Hayward RS, Tunis SR, Bass EB, Guyatt G, Evidence-Based Medicine Working Group. Users' guides to the medical literature. VIII. How to use clinical practice guidelines. B. What are the recommendations and will they help you in caring for your patients? *JAMA*. 1995;274:1630–1632.

21. Guyatt GH, Sackett DL, Sinclair JC, Evidence-Based Medicine Working Group. Users' guides to the medical literature. IX. A method for grading health care recommendations. *JAMA*. 1995;274:1800–1804.

22. Naylor CD, Guyatt GH, Evidence-Based Medicine Working Group. Users' guides to the medical literature. X. How to use an article reporting variations in the outcomes of health services. *JAMA*. 1996;275:554–558.

23. Naylor CD, Guyatt GH, Evidence-Based Medicine Working Group. Users' guides to the medical literature. XI. How to use an article about a clinical utilization review. *JAMA*. 1996;275:1435–1439.

24. Guyatt GH, Naylor CD, Juniper E, Evidence-Based Medicine Working Group. Users' guides to the medical literature. XII. How to use articles about health-related quality of life. *JAMA*. 1997;277:1232–1237.

25. Drummond MG, Richardson WS, O'Brien BJ, Levine M, Heyland D, Evidence-Based Medicine Working Group. Users' guides to the medical literature. XIII. How to use an article on economic analysis of clinical

practice. A. Are the results of the study valid? *JAMA*. 1997;277: 1552–1557.

26. O'Brien BJ, Heyland D, Richardson WS, Levine M, Drummond MF, Evidence-Based Medicine Working Group. Users' guides to the medical literature. XIII. How to use an article on economic analysis of clinical practice. B. What are the results and will they help me in caring for my patients? *JAMA*. 1997;277:1802–1806.

27. Dans AL, Dans LF, Guyatt GH, Richardson S, Evidence-Based Medicine Working Group. Users' guides to the medical literature. XIV. How to decide on the applicability of clinical trial results to your patient. *JAMA*. 1998;279:545–549.

28. Cochrane AL. Effectiveness and Efficiency. Random Reflections on Health Services. London: Nuffield Provincial Hospitals Trust, 1992.

29. Chalmers I. The Cochrane Collaboration: preparing, maintaining and disseminating systematic reviews of the effects of health care. In: Warren KS, Mosteller F, eds. Doing more good than harm: the evaluation of health care interventions. *Ann NY Acad Sc* 1993;703:156–163.

Basic Concepts

In this chapter, concepts fundamental to a review of the literature are defined. Then the structure of a typical research paper published in a scientific journal is described in order to clarify where information can be found. This chapter consists of five sections:

- ☑ Source Materials Defined
- ☑ Different Kinds of Source Materials
- ☑ Anatomy of a Scientific Paper— Finding What You Need in a Typical Research Paper
- ☑ Guidelines for a Methodological Review of the Literature
- ☑ Caroline's Quest: Learning the Concepts

SOURCE MATERIALS DEFINED

Source materials are publications and other documents about scientific knowledge that are analyzed in a review of the literature. Examples include papers published in scientific journals, reference books or chapters in books, textbooks, and reports published by governmental and nongovernmental agencies and organizations.

DIFFERENT KINDS OF SOURCE MATERIALS

Primary, Secondary, and Tertiary Source Materials

An understanding of the differences between primary, secondary, and tertiary source materials is important in selecting documents for a literature review.

- Primary source materials are original research papers written by the scientists who actually conducted the study. An example of primary source material is the description of the purpose, methods, and results section of a research paper in a scientific journal.

  A review of the scientific literature is based on the assumption that primary source materials have been examined and analyzed, unless otherwise noted. You handicap yourself if you do not use primary source materials because the details of a study may be missing from or misinterpreted in a summary about the study. Alternatively, secondary and tertiary source materials might prove to be very useful in the search for relevant primary source materials.

- Secondary source materials are papers or other documents that summarize the original work of others. In other words, secondary source materials are based on information from primary source materials. Although secondary source materials often are written by individuals other than those who actually did the research, it is possible for authors to summarize their own previously published or reported research, in which case, these later summary descriptions can still be considered secondary source materials.

Examples of secondary source materials include a summary of the literature in the introduction of each scientific research paper published in a journal, a description of what is known about a disease or treatment in a chapter in a reference book, or the synthesis you write as you review the literature.

- Tertiary source materials consist of a systematic analysis or critical review of scientific papers. The boundaries between secondary and tertiary source materials are not hard and fast; rather, they merge from one into another and differ in the degree of critical and systematic analysis as the review moves from secondary to tertiary. The term itself has not been standardized, but the generation of tertiary source materials nevertheless has become discernible over time.

The availability of tertiary source materials has evolved over the past 25 years. With the veritable explosion of scientific knowledge and the rapid rise in the number of new sources, the scientist and practitioner alike have been forced to not only stay abreast of new information, but also find more efficient ways to abstract, synthesize, and critically evaluate that knowledge. Tertiary source materials provide a variety of ways to accomplish the task of qualitative and quantitative evaluation of research findings.

Often, tertiary source materials have a specific focus. Examples include papers or articles such as a critical review of all randomized clinical trials on a subject such as the reviews in the Cochrane Library, a meta-analysis, practice guidelines, or evidence-based medicine. Each of these types of tertiary source materials is described more fully in Chapter 3.

Publications

Traditionally, source materials have been published in books or scientific journals that assume a permanence of documentation and are usually publicly accessible through libraries. This format has expanded recently to include journals published in electronic form, especially with the increased availability of the Internet. Examples of documents available on the Internet include primary source papers in peer-reviewed scientific journals and secondary source documents such as those from one of the Annual Reviews. An up-to-date list of full text journals available on the Internet can be found at http://www.ncbi. nlm.nih.gov/PubMed/fulltext.html, and a list of the Annual Reviews is given at http://biomedical. annualreviews.org/.

Regardless of how the results of a scientific study are communicated, a basic requirement of source materials is public accessibility. Not all materials that are publicly accessible are free. There may be a charge, depending on the source. Proprietary materials (those owned by individuals or organizations for their exclusive use), secret documents (such as those marked "classified" by the government), and confidential reports that cannot be accessed by people outside of a company or without a security clearance generally are not used as source materials in published, peer-reviewed journals. In other words, if you have access to such materials, but those who read your review do not, then those nonpublicly available materials probably should not be included in a review of the literature.

Peer Review

Modern scientific inquiry carries the twofold assumption that knowledge is built on previous thought, and the methods and results of research are documented and available for all to inspect and study. A basic expectation of a paper describing original research, especially in scientific journals, is that it has been evaluated through the peer-review process. A peer is a person with the same (or superior) expertise in a scientific subject as the author of a research article. A peer-reviewed paper is one that has undergone the scrutiny of one or more scientific experts. Although peer review provides one kind of quality control in the scientific process, it is not the only measure of scientific quality, nor is it a guarantee of excellence. People who read the scientific literature must decide for themselves whether each study meets the standards of the research community. A review of the literature provides one way of comparing studies and assessing the excellence of each study as well as the body of research on a specific topic.

Scientific Abstracts

A scientific abstract is an abbreviated description of a study or theory. Abstracts of papers presented at scientific meetings are considered source materials, although they usually do not include enough information about the research methods to permit a reviewer to make a judgment about the scientific merit of the study. Abstracts often are restricted in length and format, for example, no more than 250 to 500 words and usually are without citations of other research papers. For this reason, some journals, such as the *Journal of the American Medical Association*, do not permit the inclusion of references to abstracts in a summary of the review of the literature in peer-reviewed journal articles. An example of an abstract presented at a professional meeting is shown in Exhibit 2-1.

For purposes of reviewing the literature, however, abstracts of papers from scientific meetings can be useful in several ways, for example, by:

- alerting the reviewer to the more recent scientific studies,
- providing useful leads to discovering other, more fully described studies, or
- identifying the name and location of researchers who can be contacted for further information.

In many fields, abstracts of papers presented at scientific meetings are included in a special issue of the journal published by the society or organization that sponsored the meeting. Alternatively, the abstracts may be issued in booklet form at the conference. In this case, the booklet might be available only to those who attended the meeting. Contacting the author or someone who attended the meeting may be the only way of obtaining a copy of the abstracts. Recently, some pro-

Exhibit 2-1 Example of an Abstract

ANTIDEPRESSANT TREATMENT OF ELDERLY
J. Garrard, S. J. Rolnick, N. Nitz, L. Luepke,
J. Jackson, L. R. Fischer, C. Liebson, P. Bland,
R. Heinrich, L. Waller

Introduction. Since the 1980s, research has documented the underdiagnosis and undertreatment of depression in the primary care sector. Little is known about undertreatment rates of noninstitutionalized elderly. This study asked: (1) Of elderly people with an indication of depression who are living in the community, what proportion have not been treated with antidepressants (AD) during the year before or the year after the assessment? (2) What factors are associated with anti-depressant treatment during the year after assessment?

Methods. This was a longitudinal study of enrollees (N = 3,410) in an HMO that included a pharmacy benefit. All were ≥65 years and lived in noninstitutionalized settings. Subject inclusion criteria included response to the Geriatric Depression Scale (GDS) in a mail survey and 24 months continuous enrollment in the HMO (June 1992–June 1994). AD treatment one year before and after GDS screening was recorded; no feedback was provided to treating MDs. Mean age of subjects was 75 years (sd = 5.78); 62% were female.

Results. Sixteen percent of sample had an indication of depression (GDS ≥ 11) and 17% had AD use during each year; however, those treated were not necessarily those with depression. Of enrollees with GDS ≥ 11, one third had AD use during one or both years. Fifty-eight percent of enrollees with depression had no AD treatment at all. Based on logistic regression, factors associated (p < 0001) with AD treatment post-GDS included AD treatment pre-GDS (odds ratio [OR] = 25.74), gender: female (OR = 1.66), and GDS 11 (OR = 1.60); age group was not associated with AD treatment. Implications of undertreatment will be discussed.

fessional and scientific societies have begun to publish on the Internet a list of titles or abstracts of papers presented at national or international meetings. This possibility could be explored by searching the Internet for the web site of the professional society, then determining whether or not the abstracts are available. Check the list of professional societies and their web sites in Appendix A.

Citations, References, Bibliographies

A citation provides documentation about the source of an idea, statement, or research study referred to in a written document. They occur in the text or body of a scientific paper or book. In and of itself, a citation provides very little actual information; you have to go to the list of references or the bibliography (usually at the end of the paper or chapter in a book) in order to find out more about the document being cited, such as the title of the paper or the journal it was published in or the year of publication.

Different formats for citations are used, depending on the preference of the journal or book. Two common formats are numerical and author's last name. These and other examples can be found in a style manual such as *Elements of Style*.[1] Examples of the numerical and author's last name formats are shown in Exhibit 2-2.

A reference is the actual documentation of the work cited and should provide the information needed to find the paper or book or document referred to. The references of some documents, such as government reports or congressional records, are sometimes hard to decipher, and a reference librarian can be helpful in locating these materials.

Many different formats have been devised for the listing of references, and these differences have caused headaches for generations of students and researchers in the health sciences. Style manuals such as those by the American Psychological Association[2] and the American Medical Association[3] can be used.

In writing your own papers, including a review of the literature, there are also computer software programs, such as End-

Exhibit 2-2 Examples of Formats of a Citation in a Research Paper

Numerical Format: These and other examples can be found in a style manual such as *Elements of Style.*[26]
Author's Last Name Format: These and other examples can be found in a style manual such as *Elements of Style* (Strunk & White, 1979).

Note or ProCite, that can be used to automatically convert a list of references into the correct format depending on which journal you choose. Those resources are described more fully in Chapter 8. Examples of 2 of the most common formatting systems used in listing references are shown in Exhibit 2-3. These two examples, numerical and author's last name, correspond to the citations shown in Exhibit 2-2.

References for different types of documents or sources for print and electronic materials are also described on the World Wide Web (www). For example, see the following sites:

- http://library.weber.edu/libinstruct
- http://www2.gasou.edu/library/broch_ref/turabian. html/
- http://www.cs.msstate.edu/~miller/turabian.html/

Formatting rules for citations and references to printed materials are fairly well known; however, similar rules for sources on the Internet have emerged only recently. A useful web site that gives formatting guidelines for referencing Internet sources can be found at: http://www.cas.usf.edu/english/walker/mla.html/

A bibliography is like a list of references, except that it also includes references to books and other documents not quoted or cited in the text but are suggested for further reading. Authors often recommend additional materials for readers to consult if they want to develop a better understanding of the subject. Most scientific journals, however, do not encourage or

Exhibit 2-3 Examples of Formats for References

General Format:
Authors. (Year of publication). Title. Name of journal. Volume, page numbers.

Examples:
Numerical format:
26. Strunk, Jr, W & White, E B. (1979). *The Elements of Style*. NY: MacMillian Pub Co, Inc.
Author's Last Name format:
Strunk, Jr, W & White, E B. (1979). *The Elements of Style*. NY: MacMillian Pub Co, Inc.

---

allow bibliographies; these journals limit the writers to lists of references referred to in the text.

In summary, the distinctions between a citation, a reference, a list of references, and a bibliography can be described as follows:

- A citation is used in the body of a document to give credit to the publications of others (or the author's previous work).
- A reference for that citation gives complete information about where to find the materials, including the title of the scientific paper, name and volume number of the journal, and the year published.
- A list of references consists of all the references that were cited in a scientific paper and is usually given at the end of a paper or book chapter.
- A bibliography consists of not only references but also other books or papers that provide additional information about the subject being discussed. Most scientific journals restrict authors to references rather than bibliographies.

ANATOMY OF A SCIENTIFIC PAPER—FINDING WHAT YOU NEED IN A TYPICAL RESEARCH PAPER

Overview

Knowing *where* to find something is often as important as knowing what to do with it once you have found it. Thus, an understanding of the basic format or structure of a scientific paper is the first step in conducting a review of the literature.

Research articles, especially those published in scientific journals, are the most common type of source materials used in reviews of the scientific literature. Most research articles follow a standard structure, which is described in this section. By knowing this structure, you can more easily locate different parts of the research study to abstract.

In describing the 8 sections of a research paper in a typical scientific journal, some additional comments have been included that might be useful to consider.

These extra comments are set aside in boxes so they can be easily skipped by people with more experience in reading the scientific literature.

Title/Authorship Section. This section consists of the title of the paper and name and affiliations of the author or authors who conducted the research and wrote the paper.

The order of the authorship is important in most journals, with the first author usually being the person who had the most responsibility for the research study. In some fields, the most senior scientist is listed last in order of authorship. This is often the person who provided the research mentorship, the laboratory, or the grant support for the research being reported; however, he or she may not have taken the primary responsibility for the study being published. A knowledge of the field itself is needed to determine whether this protocol is followed in the peer-reviewed journals in a particular field.

Abstract Section. This section includes a brief summary of the paper. Although often identical in length and format to the abstract of a paper presented at a scientific meeting, the abstract section at the beginning of a scientific paper is just one part of the study described more fully in the remainder of the article.

Summarizing the abstract sections of journal articles does not constitute a review of the literature because there are not enough details in this brief description to allow you to understand how the research was done or how to interpret the results.

Introduction Section. Generally, this section includes 4 major parts: (1) a brief summary of the authors' review of the literature, (2) the motivation for the paper, that is, what is missing or unknown in the research literature up to this point in time, (3) an overview of the scientific theory or conceptual models on which the research was based, and (4) the purpose of the research study described in this paper. Depending on the journal or the author, the purpose of a study can be in the form of a statement, a research question, or a hypothesis.

Sometimes, authors seem to forget what their original purpose was (whether it was explicitly stated or not), especially in light of interesting results that may have answered another, unstated research question. Alternatively, authors may have satisfied the purpose they stated but then asked and answered additional research questions as the paper progresses. You have to decide for yourself whether or not the authors described a complete purpose in the introduction section of their paper and presented results about the purpose they stated in the Introduction Section.

Methods Section. Essentially a description of the procedures used to carry out the research study, this section should be complete enough to permit another researcher to replicate the study without the need to contact the authors. The methods section of a typical scientific paper includes information on methodological design, subjects, data sources, data collection methods, and statistical and analytical procedures.

Methodological Design. This describes how the research was structured, including the use of pre- and post-testing; the use of one or more groups of subjects, that is, experimental and control groups; and how subjects were assigned to these groups, for example, random assignment by the researcher or self-selection into groups by subjects of the study. This section should also include a description and definition of each of the major variables in the study, including the independent and dependent variables and the covariates. Some studies will not have an independent variable.

Subjects. This is a description of how the subjects were chosen for the study—the inclusion and exclusion criteria, sampling design, and number of subjects included in the study and their characteristics such as gender, age, disease status. This section may also include a description of how many individuals were initially selected; the number who actually participated in the study; and differences between those chosen, those who agreed to participate, those who dropped out, and those who participated at each stage of the research.

Data Sources. This section is an explanation of whether the information about the subjects in the study was based on primary source data, secondary source data, or both. Primary source data are gathered by the researchers who are reporting the study; secondary source data were gathered by others.

Secondary source data should not to be confused with secondary source materials as described at the beginning of this chapter. If secondary source data are used, then the authors should include a description of the characteristics of the database, the original reason the data were gathered, for example, for administrative records or as claims files for health care reimbursement, and the dates during which the data were gathered. Some studies will include both primary and secondary source data, for example, information from a survey of the subjects by the researchers, which the same researchers then combined with clinical data obtained from the medical charts that were recorded by the treating physicians.

Data Collection Methods. This is a description of all of the procedures used in primary source data collection to gather information from or about the subjects in the study. In this section of a journal article, the questionnaire, survey, interview protocol, or other data collection instrument will be described, including either the results of validity and reliability analyses of the data collection instrument or references to other studies that include such information.

Statistical and Analytic Procedures. This section describes the types of statistical tests or analytical procedures used and the assumptions underlying their use, if applicable.

Not all research papers published in health related journals will include these 5 subsections in a methods section, and even if they are included, they may not be in the order described above. Also, a method not described in the methods section may be mentioned later in the results section.

The choice and order of subsections in the methods section of a scientific paper depend on the field, the content, the type of study, and the choices made by the individual author.

The sudden appearance of a previously unannounced set of methods in the results or discussion section may suggest a lack of tidiness in the authors' style of reporting. Alternatively, such a practice may be entirely appropriate if the results of the main research question suggested to the researchers that they should explore something further, and the methods for that exploration are then described.

Results Section. This section gives the results of the study, and in so doing, answers the research question, verifies or refutes the hypothesis, or addresses the purposes of the study that should have been stated in the introduction section. This may be the shortest section of the entire paper, and the details may be presented concisely in one or more tables or figures.

The results section may also require the most intensive reading in order to fully understand the findings. Some journals limit this section only to results; others allow authors to discuss their interpretation of the findings in this section. If interpretations are included, you must be sure to distinguish the actual results from the authors' interpretations or opinions.

Discussion/Conclusion Section. This section usually addresses these 5 areas:

- *Summary* of the research study as it relates to the purpose or research question or hypothesis described originally.
- *Interpretation* and discussion of what these results mean. This is the part of the paper in which the authors can express their opinions about the interpretation of the findings.
- Description of the *strengths and weaknesses* of the study, including methodological strengths and weaknesses.
- Discussion of *future research*. Often the results of one study suggest additional research questions. A brief description of these topics may be included in this section of the paper.

- Statement about the *significance* of this research study on the field. This is not statistical significance, but rather a description about the impact of the findings.

As with other parts of a research paper, this discussion/ conclusion section may not include all of these topics or be in the same order, and there may also be other topics not included in this discussion.

List of References. This is a listing of all the papers or other sources cited by the authors in describing previous or related research.

Acknowledgments Section. This section includes a description of how the research study was funded, for example, the names of granting agencies or foundations, and names of individuals who assisted in the research or review.

In summary, the first step in reviewing a scientific paper in a research journal is figuring out where things are, and the 8 topics in this section provide a framework for doing that. The second step is understanding what research methods the authors used to carry out their study. The next section describes some fundamentals about research methodologies used in many of the health related journals.

GUIDELINES FOR A METHODOLOGICAL REVIEW OF THE LITERATURE

Overview

A review of the literature can be done from a number of different perspectives, such as variations in the theories on which the studies were based, the hypotheses tested, or the research results. Reviews can also include an examination of the research methodology that constitutes the framework of most empirical studies. In this section, guidelines for abstracting the research methodology of studies in the health sciences are described. Using these methodological guidelines will not only help you analyze what the authors did, but it will also let you determine what they did not do.

As described above, most papers published in scientific journals in the health and behavior literature follow a standard format: introduction, methods, results, discussion. Usually, the methods section of a journal article includes information about how the study was designed and analyzed. Exhibit 2-4 is an outline of methodological topics described in this section.

Admittedly, the list in Exhibit 2-4 may seem ambitious as a potential outline of what to abstract about the research methodology. To include all of these topics in a review of the literature, in fact, would be overkill. This is only a set of suggestions, and it is up to you to decide which are relevant to your review.

Purpose

It is best to begin by asking yourself what the purpose of the study was. Why did the authors do this particular study? What was their purpose or hypothesis or research question? Distinguish between what they said (or implied) their purpose was in the introduction section of the paper and what they actually addressed or answered in the results section.

> The authors may describe the purpose in the form of a general statement, a hypothesis, or a research question. A mark of poor research quality is a paper that does not state specifically the purpose of the study in the introduction section.

Methodology

In reviewing the methodology, consider how the authors carried out the study. For a review of elements as they are used in the social and behavioral sciences see the book by Neuman[4] and its counterpart for epidemiological research methods by

Exhibit 2-4 Methodological Topics for Reviewing Research Studies in the Health Sciences Literature

Purpose of the paper
Methodology
Research Design
- Operational Definition of Variables
- Independent and Dependent Variables
- Intervention
- Methodological Design
- Random assignment
Data Collection Instruments and Procedures
- Data Sources
- Data Collection Methods
  — Pre-post design
  — Prospective/Retrospective
  — Longitudinal/Cross-sectional
- Psychometric Characteristics of Data Collection Instruments
- Instrument Characteristics
- Standardized Instruments
- Setting
Subjects
- Unit of Analysis
- Selection Criteria
- Random Selection of Subjects
- Sampling Design
- Subject Characteristics
- Number of Subjects
  — Participation and attrition rates
  — Participant/Nonparticipant Differences
Data Analysis
- Statistical Methods
- Statistical Assumptions
Results
Discussion/Conclusion
- Interpretation of Results
- Strengths and Weaknesses
- Conclusions
References
Acknowledgments

Kleinbaum, Kupper, and Morgenstern.[5] Some major topics to consider for methodology follow.

Operational Definition of Variables. How were the variables in the study operationally defined, that is, what procedures or steps did the researchers use to measure the variables of interest? For example, how did they operationally define health or quality of life or education?

Independent and Dependent Variables. Specify the independent and dependent variables. Describe the independent variable in terms of what was actually done to the experimental group (the intervention in some studies) and to the control group.

Intervention. Describe the procedures or treatment applied to one or more of the groups of subjects, usually to the experimental group, including the timing of the procedures with respect to data collection. Sometimes these intervention procedures are summarized as part of the methodological design.

Depending on the purpose of the research, some studies may not include an actual intervention. Alternatively, the intervention may be some external event, such as a change in health policy or a formulary change, and the purpose of the study is to examine the effects of such a change. In these kinds of studies, the author is expected to give a clear description of the "externally applied" intervention. Sometimes such a description is not given because it is so well known in the field; if this is the case, there should be at least a reference to a book or journal article or other document or source material that does describe the well-known intervention.

An example of an intervention is a diabetes education program presented to the experimental subjects but not to those in the control group. Sometimes interventions are not applied by the researchers themselves. For example, an intervention might be a federal regulation such as a restriction on the use of antipsychotic medications in nursing homes. In this example, the nursing homes in the experimental group may have been under the federal regulation and those in the comparison group of homes may not be operating under the regulation.

Methodological Design. What was the study design? In the behavioral sciences, the four major designs include experimental, quasi-experimental, pre-experimental, or observational. In epidemiological terms, similar designs are used but are described in different terms. Some examples include randomized control trials, case-control studies, cohort designs, and descriptive designs. Qualitative designs would also be listed here.

See the texts by Campbell and Stanley[6] and Cook and Campbell[7] for a description of the behavioral sciences designs. Kleinbaum, Kupper, and Morgenstern[5] describe the epidemiological designs.

For example, did the researchers use focus groups,[8] or the Delphi technique, or an interview protocol that they developed?

Random Assignment. How were the subjects of the study assigned to the experimental and control groups? If the assignment was random, then "random assignment" was used. If subjects could choose for themselves which groups to be in, or if they were already in groups to begin with (such as smokers and nonsmokers), then random assignment was not used.

Technically the term *experimental design* implies the use of random assignment of subjects to groups, but recent usage has become a bit lax. You need to ask yourself whether or not the authors specifically said that the subjects were "randomized," or randomly assigned, if they said they used an experimental design. A general rule of thumb is that if the authors knew enough about methodological designs to randomly assign subjects to groups, then they should have known enough to brag about it in the methodology section.

Also, bear in mind that there is a big difference between random assignment and random sampling. The purpose of random assignment is to create 2 or more subject groups that are as equal as possible at the beginning of an experimental study; usually, one of these groups is designated as the experimental group, the other is the control group. Random assignment is a methodological design issue. Random sampling is concerned with the selection of a representative sample of subjects from a population.

Data Collection Instruments and Procedures

This group of topics is concerned with how information was collected. Some basic reference books that might be useful include those on questionnaire design,[9] conducting a survey,[10] and the design and use of focus groups.[8]

Data Sources. As described earlier in this chapter, primary source data consist of information gathered by the researchers who conducted the original study from subjects in that study. Alternatively, data gathered by others or for purposes other than research are called secondary source data.

Secondary source data can come in many forms. Some examples include information gathered for administrative purposes (for example, in registering people when they are admitted to a hospital) or for reimbursement of health care services or to document the effects of treatment. If secondary source data were used, note why the data were collected initially, for example, health services claims files or as part of administrative records.

Another example of secondary source data gathered for purposes other than research includes information collected about a patient's symptoms by clinicians in a medical center and recorded in a clinical record. If a researcher is interested in using that information in a study of those patients, then he or she would be using secondary source data. On the other hand, if the researcher surveys the patients directly about their symptoms, then the data would be primary source data.

An example of a national secondary source dataset is the National Health and Nutrition Examination Survey (NHANES), which is a national survey of Americans conducted 3 times over the past 15 years by the National Center for Health Statistics.

Data Collection Methods. Begin by noting when the data were collected, for example, "pre-post-post" for one pretesting and two post-testings. Also determine whether the data were gathered prospectively or retrospectively. Were the data gathered at 2 or more points in time (possibly a longitudinal study) or at a single point in time (cross-sectional)? If primary source data were used, what specific data collection methods or instruments were used to collect information? For example, was the information gathered by questionnaire, survey, telephone or in-person interview?

Psychometric Characteristics of Data Collection Instruments. For each data collection instrument, note whether or not the author describes results of validity and reliability testing of the data collection instrument. If the instruments were developed by the author, but no information is given about validity and reliability, then make a note of the lack of information about these fundamental psychometric characteristics.

In the language of data collection, an "instrument" can be a questionnaire or a list of interview questions, sometimes called a "protocol," or a set of instructions for recording certain behaviors of subjects by the person observing those subjects. For example, a questionnaire might consist of questions about different kinds of foods, and the subject is asked to check off each food he or she ate. An interview protocol is generally a set of questions that the researcher asks. The wording and the order of the questions are both important, and the interviewer usually is not allowed to deviate from that order.

Psychometrics is the study of the characteristics of tests or data collection instruments, including the validity and reliability of the instrument. Validity concerns whether the data collection instrument measures what it was intended to measure. Reliability generally is concerned with stability over time. If researchers want to measure change in the health of a group of subjects, then they do not want an instrument that varies, either in the way it is used or interpreted (validity) or in its consistency each time it is used (reliability).

Instrument Characteristics. Other basic characteristics about a data collection instrument might include the number of items or questions or the average time needed to gather the information from individual subjects. If the instrument was a survey, note whether or not the data were collected by mail or telephone.

Some journals permit the author to publish an author-developed survey as an appendix at the end of the journal article; if such a survey has been included, indicate this in your notes.

Standardized Instruments. If the instruments were standardized, what references are given about this standardization?

What normative groups were used in the original standardization, and did the subjects in this study have the same or similar characteristics as those in the normative group? For example, the norms for a questionnaire about food preferences may have been based on responses from people living in rural Minnesota, but such norms would probably not be appropriate for Chinese Americans living in San Francisco.

Setting. If relevant to the area of research being reviewed, note the setting in which the data were collected, for example, urban or rural, community, hospital, or nursing home, home or school.

Subjects

Summarize the key features about the subjects of the research study.

Unit of Analysis. What was the unit of analysis? Generally, there are 4 choices: individual, group, organization, and social artifact.

Examples of the different units of analysis are the following:
- Individual. The subject of the study is an individual person. For example, in a study of smoking behavior of teenage children each child would be a unit of analysis.
- Group. The subject is a group of people. For example, in a study of the relationship between family size and group cohesiveness, each family would be considered the unit of analysis.
- Organization. The subject is an organization such as a health department or school or hospital. For example, a study of health departments throughout the United States that do or do not have staff assigned to develop prevention programs for AIDS would use the health department as its unit of analysis.

- Social artifact. A social artifact has been defined in the research literature as the product of a social being. Examples of social artifacts include a health care policy or a law or practice guideline. An example of research in which a social artifact was the subject would be a study of the characteristics of state guidelines on vaccination of preschool children. Thus the state guideline (which is a social artifact) from each of 50 states would be the unit of analysis for this study.

Most, but not all, studies in the health and behavioral sciences use the individual as the unit of analysis. If another unit of analysis was used, then it is important to determine how the researchers operationally defined that unit. For example, if an organization, such as a hospital, was the unit of analysis, then did the researchers define what they meant by a hospital in terms such as bed size, geographic area, or type of ownership?

Selection Criteria. What were the inclusion and exclusion criteria used to select subjects?

An example of inclusion criteria might be age range and type of health plan: only people between the ages of 18 and 64 and who were enrolled in a managed health care organization qualified for this study. Thus, people whose ages were below 18 or above 64 and/or those who had some other kind of health care plan were excluded from the study.

Random Selection and Sampling Design. How were subjects selected for this study? Did the researcher select the subjects and did he or she select them randomly from a population of potential subjects? If the subjects volunteered for the study, then they were not randomly selected. These are very important points to note since the generalization of results to a population is not technically possible without random selection.

Under this topic, you should also note which sampling design was used. Some examples include simple random sample, stratified random sample, cluster sample, and convenience sample.

Sometimes researchers do not describe the sampling design they used. Read the article carefully to see if you can figure this out from their description of what they did. An excellent book on sampling designs is the one by Kish.[11]

Subject Characteristics. Which subject characteristics were described by the authors? Examples include gender, age (recorded as mean age or percent within age categories or age range), race or ethnicity, or other characteristics such as disease status, geographic location, or socio-economic status.

Number of Subjects. How many subjects were in the study? The number of subjects in a study is often abbreviated as (N =) in tables of results.

The number of subjects is a fundamental piece of information that some authors fail to provide; therefore, you might consider noting the total number or its absence in every study. If there is more than one group of subjects, for example, an experimental (E) group and a control (C) group, then record the number for each group in this cell, for example: E (N = 126), C (N = 140).

Summarizing the number of subjects can involve a number of related questions that may be important to your review of the literature.

Participation and Attrition Rates. What was the total number of subjects the researchers began with, compared to the number who left during the study, and the final number of subjects who completed the study? These enumerations are sometimes surprisingly difficult to find in a scientific paper.

Participant/Nonparticipant Differences. What information was given about differences between people who stayed in the study and those who either refused to be in the study in the first place or left before the study ended? A similar discussion about participant and nonparticipant differences might be in terms of the dropout rate or respondent and nonrespondent analysis.

Equally noteworthy is the absence of a description of such differences. This is an important issue that concerns the possibility of bias in the final group of subjects for whom data were analyzed.

Data Analysis

Summarize how the data were analyzed, including the use of descriptive statistics such as percentages or means, a bivariate analysis such as chi-square or *t* test, or multivariate techniques such as analysis of variance or regression analysis.

A basic statistics textbook is a good resource in providing background material for this section. The classic book by Siegel on nonparametric statistics is also useful.[12,13] Statistical methods commonly used in the epidemiological literature include those described in books by Fleiss[14] and Kahn & Sempos.[15]

Statistical Methods. What specific statistical and other analytic procedures were used in the study, for example, logistic regression, analysis of variance, factor analysis, path analysis? An example of an analytic technique for qualitative research would be a content analysis of interview data.

Statistical Assumptions. What assumptions (or violation of assumptions) were made by the author about the use of the analytic techniques, other than the usual procedures described in introductory texts?

Results

In analyzing the results of a study, ask yourself the following questions:

- Did the authors answer the research question they posed in the introduction section of the paper? After you have read the entire paper, ask whether this was the right question in the first place.
- Did the authors provide an answer to a research question that they did not ask initially? In other words, did some results creep into the paper without an explicit research question being described? Were these additional research questions appropriate to the study?

A transition from one research question or purpose to another can sometimes be detected in the results section or, more often, in the discussion section of the paper. Such a change usually occurs because the authors allowed the statistically significant results to dictate the hypothesis rather than the other way around. Differences between initial and later research questions may be important to note in a review of the study.

Discussion/Conclusion

This collection of topics describes the authors' scientific opinions about the study. In reviewing a paper, you need to separate the results of the study, which are facts, from the authors' interpretations or opinions of the results and their significance.

Interpretation of Results. As a reviewer, it is up to you to decide whether the authors' interpretations are logical and valid based on the results of the study. You must also decide whether or not the results of this study are consistent with the findings of other studies on the same topic as described elsewhere in the literature.

Strengths and Weaknesses. What strengths and weaknesses of the study were described? Specifically, did the authors address issues such as whether the findings could be generalized, problems with methodological design that were present but could not have been remedied, sample size adequacy, or sampling design?

> Authors who do not point out the weaknesses of their own studies make themselves vulnerable to such criticisms from others. Most authors are pleased to describe the strengths of their studies; they may be a bit reluctant to discuss the weaknesses.

Conclusions. When reviewing this section, describe what the authors concluded from this study. Note especially whether or not the conclusions and the significance of the findings related to the results. Do you agree with those conclusions?

Caroline's Quest: Learning the Concepts

"So," Caroline looked at Professor Dickerson somewhat challengingly, "isn't the Matrix Method just simply a spreadsheet that's called a Review Matrix?"

"No," he replied, "there's more to it than that. The Matrix Method is a system for how you can access, integrate, and use information from a variety of sources in order to prepare a written synthesis of the scientific literature. In the past, researchers could keep up with the current literature by reading several journals or monitoring the work of a few, well-known scientists in a field, or they could simply call or write their friends who did research in that area."

"What's wrong with doing that now?" Caroline asked. This business of accessing and integrating and so forth was beginning to sound rather time-consuming, as she thought about all the other things she had to do to get her thesis completed. She asked, "Why bother?"

Professor Dickerson looked over his glasses at her and said dryly, "Because the amount of scientific literature has grown tremendously. It's rarely possible to develop a comprehensive understanding about the research literature on a topic by using such informal methods. Fortunately, more advanced tools for searching and accessing the literature have become available over the past decade or so. The Matrix Method takes advantage of those tools."

"But, no one else in my program has to go to all this trouble for their lit reviews." Caroline's voice verged on the edge of a whine, "They just go to the library, read a few articles, and write up a summary. Takes them several days at most."

Professor Dickerson nodded his head, "Yes, anyone can do a sloppy job, Caroline." He looked over the top of his glasses at her. "But they run the risk of not understanding the literature — not the depth nor the full scope of what's out there. Furthermore, they could miss some of the more important articles or even major trends in a field of research. It is also the case that whatever they write, whether it's a thesis, a scientific paper, or whatever, has to withstand the scrutiny of readers who are likely to know the literature quite well. . . . like your thesis committee members."

Caroline's eyes were beginning to glaze over as he continued, "The person who does a cursory literature review could find himself doing what he thinks is original research, only to discover at the end that that very study was done and reported previously by someone else."

Professor Dickerson's enthusiasm began to build. "The process of doing a thorough review of the literature is analogous to solving a mystery. If you miss some of the important clues, then you may not ever find out who or what was responsible for the crime — or what the study really meant, in this case. The Matrix Method gives you a systematic way to lay out all the pieces and put the puzzle together."

He looked at her with a grin. "The effort will pay off for you, Caroline. You'll see. Now, let's get started."

Under Professor Dickerson's direction, Caroline set up a 3-ring binder with 4 sections. She further subdivided the first section, Paper Trail, into 5 parts, with one page, to begin with, for each part. The different sections and subsections of Caroline's Lit Review Book are shown in Exhibit 2-5.

She then went to the biomedical library to begin by looking up some reference books on smoking behavior.

Exhibit 2-5 Outline of Caroline's Lit Review Book for Her Thesis Topic

---

Paper Trail
- Keywords
- Key Sources
- Electronic Bibliographic Database
- Internet
- Notes

Documents Section

Review Matrix

Synthesis

REFERENCES

1. Strunk W, White EB. *Elements of Style.* New York: Macmillan; 1979.
2. American Psychological Association. *Publication Manual of the American Psychological Association.* 4th ed. Washington, DC; 1994.
3. Iverson C. *American Medical Association Manual of Style: A Guide for Authors and Editors.* 9th ed. Baltimore, MD. Williams & Wilkins; 1998.
4. Neuman WL. *Social Research Methods: Qualitative and Quantitative Approaches.* 3rd ed. Boston: Allyn & Bacon; 1997.
5. Kleinbaum DG, Kupper LL, Morgenstern H. *Epidemiologic Research: Principles and Quantitative Methods.* New York: Van Nostrand Reinhold; 1982.
6. Krueger RA. *Focus Groups: A Practical Guide for Applied Research.* Thousand Oaks, CA: Sage Publications; 1994.
7. Campbell DT, Stanley JC. *Experimental and Quasi-Experimental Designs for Research.* Chicago: Rand McNally; 1966.
8. Cook TD, Campbell DT. *Quasi-Experimentation: Design and Analysis Issues for Field Settings.* Chicago: Rand McNally; 1979.
9. Salant P, Dilman DA. *How to Conduct Your Own Survey.* New York: John Wiley & Sons; 1994.
10. Dillman DA. *Mail and Telephone Surveys: The Total Design Method.* New York: John Wiley & Sons; 1978.
11. Kish L. *Survey Sampling.* New York: John Wiley & Sons; 1995.
12. Siegel S. *Nonparametric Statistics for the Behavioral Sciences.* New York: McGraw-Hill; 1956.
13. Siegel S, Castellan NJJ. *Nonparametric Statistics for the Behavioral Sciences.* 2d ed. New York: McGraw-Hill; 1988.
14. Fleiss JL. *Statistical Methods for Rates and Proportions.* New York: John Wiley & Sons; 1981.
15. Kahn HA, Sempos, CT. Statistical Methods in Epidemiology. (*Monographs in Epidemiology and Biostatistics*, Vol. 12). New York: Oxford University Press; 1989.

The Matrix
Method

Paper Trail: How To Plan and Manage a Search of the Literature

This chapter discusses how to set up and use a Paper Trail and how to organize and conduct a search for source materials in your review of the literature. The five sections of this chapter are the following:

☑ What Is a Paper Trail?
☑ How To Create a Paper Trail
☑ How To Find Source Materials: Creating and Using a Paper Trail
☑ Tips on Searching for Source Documents
☑ Caroline's Quest: Managing the Search

WHAT IS A PAPER TRAIL?

For purposes of the Matrix Method, a Paper Trail is a record of lists and notes to help in planning and in keeping track of what you have done as you review the literature on a particular topic; it is a method of documenting your search for relevant materials.

Advantages of a Paper Trail for You

A Paper Trail is both a map of where you are going and a diary of where you have been in your search for source documents. The map gets you started and buys you efficiency; the diary helps you remember what you have done so you can avoid redoing the same thing. Even people with a prodigious memory will inevitably find themselves backtracking and trying to relocate materials if they have not taken the time to make a list of the sources explored and the articles considered. It is also useful to write down the names of people who were (or were not) helpful. A knowledgeable and enthusiastic librarian can be worth his or her weight in gold—write down the person's name for future reference. The same advice applies to helpful faculty and colleagues.

HOW TO CREATE A PAPER TRAIL

Getting Organized

Just as you unfold a map as the first step in going on a hike in unfamiliar territory, the first step in beginning a review of the literature should be to set up a Paper Trail section in your Lit Review Book. At its simplest, a pencil-and-paper trail will suffice. Although index cards may be traditional, they are not as useful in the Matrix Method as standard notebook paper or a computer. If you don't have a computer available, then take some notebook paper on every visit to the library in order to record notes. At the end of the day, put them in your Paper Trail section. Even if you use a word processor, it is useful to store a printout of that information for your Paper Trail section. In the interests of simplicity, a paper version will be described here, which can be converted to a word processor.

Set up a Paper Trail Section

Begin by setting up the Paper Trail Section with 5 parts, each with some blank paper for making notes:

1. **Key Words**

   A key word is a term or phase that describes a research topic. In this subsection keep a list of key words you have used as well as others you have considered but discarded.

   Begin the Key Words subsection by writing down the purpose of this review of the literature at the top of the page. Think of the words that describe that topic. For example, if it is a review of the literature on the epidemiology of pneumonia, some of the key words might be: *pneumonia, nursing homes, elderly.*

   As you collect information during the literature review, add to this list. Some of the terms considered initially may not be useful as the literature review progresses. Leave these terms on the list, but draw a line through them—it is useful to know which terms did not work as well as those that did.

2. **Key Sources**

   This is another list that consists of the names of reference books, journals, government reports, and other materials that you considered or reviewed. The same logic of maintaining a list of where you're going and where you've been applies to all the library sources considered or explored. For example, in the Key Sources part of the Paper Trail section, create a page (on paper or computer) and keep a running list of reference books, other books, journals, other print sources, bookmarks on the World Wide Web (www), and electronic bibliographic databases.

3. **Electronic Bibliographic Databases**
   In this section, make a list of electronic databases used, such as MEDLINE, CancerLit, and HealthSTAR. What were the search strategies? Include the key words used, as well as restrictions on the search, such as English language journals only or review articles only. Include the period of time covered, for example, 1965 to the present. Insert in this section a copy of the results of searches of the electronic bibliographic databases, such as MEDLINE, including the search strategies used to generate the list of references.

4. **Internet**
   When researching on the Web, it is easy to lose track of what has been explored unless you keep a record. Do that in this subsection. Also, set a bookmark of the Universal Resource Locator (URL) for commonly used web sites. Another possibility is to print the home page of a web site and put it in this section of your Paper Trail.

5. **Notes**
   This is a miscellaneous subsection in the Paper Trail. Treat it like a running diary of things that you need to remember. Make notes about where to find hard-to-locate materials, for example, "Journal of Scientific Wonder is located in the third stack from the left in the basement of the library of the county medical examiner." The notes refer to the search process, not the papers themselves.

   Also use this subsection to record additional references of scientific papers or other source materials discovered in the process of looking at other sources. Put a check mark by each as you read and accept it or discard it. In recording a reference, use a standard format in order to make sure you have all needed information, including publishers, dates, and page numbers. Inevitably, the one article without the year of publication will be the very one that is essential in your synthesis of the literature. It is best to be consistent in the first place. Examples of standard formats are shown in Chapter 2, choose the reference format of a journal you use frequently.

In recording a reference to a paper in a journal, consider the following tip. Scientific journals are expensive to produce, and editors are inclined to be stingy with space. One way some publishers have of saving space in the references section of a book or journal article is to restrict the names of multiple authors to the first 3 individuals followed by et al. for the remaining authors. In reviewing these papers, however, you might want to depart from this protocol by writing down the names of all of the authors. There is a practical reason for going to this extra effort. In many fields of study, the research is conducted jointly by a number of scientists. Although the first author of a paper presumably had the most responsibility for writing the paper or doing the study, some of the other authors may have been publishing in the field over a longer period of time. These more established scientists sometimes are listed last in the authorship.

Alternatively, authors of some large, well-established research teams have chosen to list their names alphabetically, signifying equal importance in the contribution of all members of the research team to the study. With either practice, there can be a problem in tracking the work of specific individuals if the format of the reference is limited to the first 3 authors, followed by et al. Consider recording all of the authors' names; usually they are listed on the paper itself. Once the Paper Trail section is set up, you are ready to begin your search of the literature.

HOW TO FIND SOURCE MATERIALS:
CREATING AND USING A PAPER TRAIL

Reference Books: Learn Something about the Topic

If you are not familiar with the area or subject of the literature you are reviewing, it is important to take time to learn some of the fundamental information about the disease or issue. Reference books can be especially useful resources at the beginning of a review of the literature in providing an overview of the topic, as well as a potential list of key words. In a biomedical library, these books are often kept on reserve and therefore are readily available. Check with the reference librarian about the major reference books on the topic you want to review. For example, if you are reviewing the literature on treatment of arthritis, then consult a basic medical textbook about arthritic conditions and their treatments before conducting a review of the research literature on arthritis medications.

As you consult a reference or textbook, develop a list of key words, including the terms those authors used. Maintain a list of the textbooks or reference books examined, and with each, record references of papers and other books mentioned at the end of chapters that relate to your subject. Alternatively, photocopy these source materials and put them in the Notes subsection of the Paper Trail section. Record the names of journals cited frequently in these source materials, whether or not any of the papers are of specific interest. This list of frequently appearing journals will also be useful in the next step: collecting articles from the scientific journals.

If you are already familiar with the subject under review, the most efficient approach might be to launch the search for source documents using your list of key words to run a computer search.

Key Words: Accessing Electronic Databases

Key words are terms that describe the characteristics of the subject you are reviewing. They are especially useful in searching electronic databases for documents on specific topics.

Standardized and Nonstandardized Key Words. Some databases use a standardized list of key words; others do not. A standardized or structured set of key words is established by the organization that manages the electronic database, and users generally are restricted to those words in searching the database. In a database that allows the use of nonstandardized key words, users can use whatever terms they wish.

Two examples of electronic databases are MEDLINE and Current Contents. MEDLINE, which covers a wide array of journals in the health sciences, uses a list of standardized key words that is updated and published annually by the National Library of Medicine.

MEDLINE key words are available in a book, the *Medical Subject Headings: Annotated Alphabetical List,* and the list is known as MeSH headings. This book is available in most biomedical research libraries. A description of MeSH headings can also be found on the Internet at http://www.nlm.nih.gov/mesh/mesh-home.html/. An electronic form of MeSH headings also exists in some interface packages with the on-line bibliographic referencing systems.

Despite having a structured system, in practice, MEDLINE maps your terms onto its standardized key words, thus the database is more user-friendly than you might expect. By using the standardized MeSH headings as key words, you may buy yourself greater precision in searching the literature.

Although Current Contents does not require the use of a set of standardized key words, this lack of a structured list can create other problems. The terms you think of may not be those chosen by the researchers, or they may not be used consistently throughout the field. Thus you may miss finding an important document or study because you did not think of the key word that others used to index that article.

Key Words Available in Abstracts

Another source of key words or terms can be found in the abstracts available in electronic bibliographic databases. The list of key words may differ, depending on whether the electronic database uses a standardized or nonstandardized set of terms. For example, consider different abstracts of the same paper described in MEDLINE and Current Contents. In the MEDLINE abstract, shown in Exhibit 3-1, the key words are listed under the heading: MeSH Subject Headings. Note that 2 of the 23 MeSH subject headings have an asterisk, *Medication Systems and *Residential Facilities. Within a MEDLINE abstract, an asterisk by a MeSH heading indicates the primary focus of a paper. To find other papers that had a primary focus on those topics, you would restrict your MEDLINE search to those asterisked MeSH headings.

Exhibit 3-1 A MEDLINE Abstract

Unique Identifier
98094391
Authors
Garrard J., Cooper SL., Goertz C.
Title
Drug use management in board and care facilities
Source
Gerontologist. 37(6):748–56, 1997 Dec.
MeSH Subject Headings

Activities of Daily Living	Interviews
Age Factors	Long-Term Care
Aged	Male
Attention Deficit and	*Medication Systems
Mental Disorders	Behavior Disorders
Attitude of Health Personnel	Mental Retardation
Comparative Study	Prescriptions, Drug
Data Interpretation, Statistical	Psychotropic Drugs/ad
Disabled Persons	(Administration & Dosage)
Drug Storage	Questionnaires
Female	*Residential Facilities
Frail Elderly	Support, Non-U.S. Gov't
Human	

Abstract
The purpose of this study was to describe medication management in board and care facilities throughout Minnesota. A triangulation of data collection methods was used, including mail questionnaires (N = 98 facilities), telephone interviews (N = 64 facilities), and site visits (N = 15 facilities). Major issues

---

continues

Exhibit 3-1 continued

examined included characteristics of board and care facilities, staffing, residents, and drug management systems. Results showed that staff in 86% of the board and care facilities surveyed provided medication storage, 83% gave medication reminders, and 69% administered medications to one or more residents. Site visits revealed a wide diversity in the characteristics of managers and their attitudes toward medication administration.

Publication Type
Journal Article.

Language
English

In the Current Contents abstract, the key words are listed in 2 sections: Author Key words, with 4 terms that the authors suggested when they submitted the paper to the journal and an additional section, Key Words Plus, which Current Contents staff added.

There are also subtle differences between the MEDLINE and Current Contents key words for the same article. The 23 terms in the MEDLINE list are more comprehensive than the set of 4 terms the authors provided, as listed in the Current Contents abstract in Exhibit 3-2. (Although unrelated to the key words, another difference between the 2 databases is the provision of an address for the authors in the Current Contents system, but not in the MEDLINE system. Thus, if you wanted to contact an author of a paper, then that information is available in the Current Contents abstract, but not in the MEDLINE abstract.)

In general, once you find an abstract on an electronic database that is a good example of the topic under review, use those key words to search the database for related articles or

Exhibit 3-2 A Current Contents® Abstract

Authors
Garrard J., Cooper SL., Goertz C.
Title
Drug use management in board and care facilities
Source
Gerontologist. 37(6):748–756, 1997 Dec.
Author Keywords
Board and care facilities   Medication management
Psychotropic drugs   Long-term care
KeyWords Plus
Homes
Abstract
The purpose of this study was to describe medication management in board and care facilities throughout Minnesota. A triangulation of data collection methods was used, including mail questionnaires (N = 98 facilities), telephone interviews (N = 64 facilities), and site visits (N = 15 facilities). Major issues examined included characteristics of board and care facilities, staffing, residents, and drug management systems. Results showed that staff in 86% of the board and care facilities surveyed provided medication storage, 83% gave medication reminders, and 69% administered medications to one or more residents. Site visits revealed a wide diversity in the characteristics of managers and their attitudes toward medication administration. (References: 14)
Language
English
Publication Type
Article
CC Categories
Public health & health care science
Subset
Current Contents/Social & Behavioral Sciences

---

continues

Exhibit 3-2 continued

Institution
Reprint available from:
Garrard J
UNIV MINNESOTA
SCH PUBL HLTH
INST HLTH SERV RES
BOX 729
420 DELAWARE ST SE
MINNEAPOLIS, MN 55455
USA

Courtesy of Institute for Scientific Information, Philadelphia, Pennsylvania.

---

papers. An informed reference librarian can also be a good resource in planning an advanced search strategy.

Electronic Bibliographic Databases: A Computer Search of the Literature

Once you have generated some key words, whether or not the list is complete, consider running a computer search of the literature using an electronic bibliographic database such as Current Contents or MEDLINE. There is a growing number of electronic bibliographic databases available that vary by subject and period of time covered, some of which are listed in Exhibit 3-3. Some of these databases are available free of charge on the Internet. For example, since June 1997, the National Library of Medicine has provided free access to MEDLINE on the Internet through 2 sites, PubMed and Internet Grateful Med. Differences in these 2 sites and how to use each can be found at http://www.index.nlm.nih.gov/databases/freemedl.html/.

In running an initial search of the literature on an electronic database, use a search strategy that is as broad as possible. For example, when specifying the instructions for an electronic search, include all types of papers, such as editorials or review summaries or letters to the editor, about a particular scientific topic. Even if you do not intend to use such nonempirical communications in your final review of the literature, they may be useful in locating other, more relevant scientific papers that you might not have found otherwise. Editorials and let-

---

Exhibit 3-3 Electronic Bibliographic Databases in the Health Sciences

Database	Dates Included	Subjects Covered
Bioethicsline	1973–present	Ethics in health care and medical research
CancerLit	1983–present	Cancer research including abstracts from scientific meetings
CINAHL	1982–present	Nursing and allied health
Current Contents	Period varies	Multidisciplinary
Dissertation Abstracts	1861–present	Abstracts of masters and doctoral dissertations from North American universities
Health and Psychosocial Instruments	1985–present	Measurement instruments in health related and behavioral sciences
HealthSTAR	1975–present	Health services, technology, administration, and research
International Pharmaceutical Abstracts	1970–present	Drug therapy and pharmacy practice
MEDLINE	1966–present	Health sciences
PsycLit or Psyc INFO	1974–present	Psychological literature
Sociological Abstracts/ Social Planning	1963–present	Sociological literature

ters to the editor can also be enlightening in suggesting counterpoints or alternative opinions about a study.

Maintain a copy of database search strategies, that is, the instructions you specify for the electronic search, as well as the complete list of source materials selected. A practical way to do this is to copy the instructions just before initiating the electronic search, then either store the information in a computer file or print out the instructions and keep it in the Electronic Bibliographic Databases subsection of your Paper Trail. This information may be useful when you check the thoroughness of your search.

A few words of caution. First, conduct the computer search of the literature yourself. Don't depend solely on a reference librarian because there are many decisions to be made during the search about which articles to select. Running a computer search yourself will give you the opportunity to scan a title, consider which authors were involved in the study, or rapidly read the abstract. This information may be crucial in deciding whether or not to select the article for further consideration. Furthermore, with the right kind of computer facilities, you can run your own database search in the middle of the night when most reference librarians are not available.

In the process of a computer search, you will begin to pick up subtle cues about what else is in the literature. For example, when scrolling through a list of abstracts by a particular author, you will notice the names of other authors associated with a topic or a journal that often publishes papers in this area. Such information is useful in the later stages of the literature review. More importantly, by running a computer search yourself, you know exactly what was done and which decisions you made to arrive at a specific list of scientific books and journal articles.

A second cautionary note is to remember that not all journals are included in even the most frequently used databases such as MEDLINE. This is true especially for some of the newer journals or those with a specialized focus. For this reason, it's important to extend your search of the literature to the print versions of some of the scientific journals.

Scientific Journals:
The Most Current Research Literature

If your goal is to generate a list of journal articles related to a specific topic, consider going to the research library and scanning the titles of articles in the annual indexes of specific journals. Most journals provide such a list of all papers published during the preceding year. These annual indexes usually can be found in the last issue of each year. Some journals index papers by topics, and key words can be used efficiently by locating relevant articles under those topics. Record the references of each study related to your key words.

Be efficient. Begin with the annual index of recent journals and work backwards in time: 1999, then 1998, then 1997, and so forth. This strategy is useful because the more recent papers will provide references to papers published previously, and you can build your list of references by going to those already discovered by those authors.

An alternative strategy would be to take each issue of each journal and scan the table of contents. This is useful for the most recent journals that do not yet have an annual index. With either approach, if an article is specifically related to your literature review, read it quickly and decide whether or not it is one to keep. If so, make a photocopy of that paper, including the references section of the study (the references section of a paper is one of the *most* important parts of any paper or source material that you photocopy). Look at the beginning (often at the bottom of the abstract of the paper) or at the end of the article to see if key words are given. Record these in your key words list and use them to search for other materials. Put whatever photocopies of articles you make in the Documents section of your Lit Review Book. This is covered in detail in the next chapter.

An electronic alternative to scanning the titles of journals in the library is to use UnCover®, developed by the Colorado Association of Research Libraries (CARL). CARL's web site is: http://uncweb.carl.org/. UnCover is a searchable database of current article information taken from more than 17,000 journals published since fall 1988. Users can perform key word and author searches from the tables of contents of most scientific and health professional journals; new journals are added to the database within several days of publication. The search feature of UnCover is free. The company also provides a document delivery service for which there is a charge.

Government Reports: How To Find Them

Over the past 5 or more years, different health-related agencies of the federal government have begun to provide special reports on the Internet. A free, searchable database of documents printed by the U. S. Government Printing Office (GPO) is available on the Internet at GPO Access. The web site is: http://www.access.gpo.gov/. The Users' Guide for GPO Access is located at http://www.access.gpo.gov/su_docs/dbsearch. html/.

Discuss with a reference librarian the search procedures for accessing congressional reports and other federal documents. Many of these materials are not research reports, nor are they necessarily peer-reviewed even if they are reports of scientific studies. These documents can be very useful, however, in gathering background material about a topic or issue and suggesting other sources to include in your review of the literature.

An additional Internet resource available on GPO Access is the Government Information Locator Service (GILS), which is a web site for finding publicly available federal information resources, including electronic information resources. A brief description of GILS can be found at http://www.access.gpo.gov/su_docs/gils/whatgils.html/, and the GILS web site is http://www.access.gpo.gov/su_docs/gils/gils.html/.

One of the more general, nongovernmental resources on the Internet for searching for government publications and databases on national and international web sites is the Virtual Reference Desk at: http://www.virtualref.com/. This site was developed and is maintained by a reference librarian.

Critical Evaluations of the Literature: Critiques by Experts

Increasingly, researcher and practitioner alike are faced with the problem of not only staying abreast of what is new, but also critically evaluating and integrating the results across multiple studies. Although there is no universally agreed upon system for synthesizing research studies, different ways of coping with the information explosion have been developed over the past few decades. Four of these strategies are described in this section: (1) review articles, (2) meta-analysis, (3) practice guidelines, and (4) the Cochrane Library.

All 4 are examples of tertiary source information, as described in Chapter 2; however, there are some major differences among them—some are qualitative, others quantitative; some are guidelines for practitioners, others are tools for researchers; some are locally focused, others are international in scope. What they represent, however, are resources that can be explored as you review the literature. Be aware of their existence and consider using them as adjuncts to the usual electronic bibliographic databases.

Review Articles. In general, a review summarizes or synthesizes what is new or currently known about a topic. Some review articles also provide a critical analysis of the research methods and the quality of the research. Reviews can be found in a variety of print and electronic sources. Some peer-reviewed journals that concentrate on original or primary source papers will periodically publish a review article, such as the 1995 paper, "Alcohol and mortality: a review," which was published in the *Journal of Clinical Epidemiology.*[1] In many fields, there are also journals, such as the *Epidemiological Review,* that publish only review articles. Finally, there is a series of *Annual Reviews* that has been published since 1932. Currently, there are 27 volumes; see a list of these volumes in Appendix A. Further information about these and future volumes can be found at http://www.annualreviews.org/.

Even reviews need to be read critically.[2, 3] There is a growing literature on criteria for evaluating the quality of reviews for researchers,[3] practitioners,[2] and science writers.[4] In addition, checklists have been developed for what constitutes an acceptable review in the health sciences.[5] An example of a critical review of the quality of reviews in epidemiology is a paper published in 1998, "Quality of reviews in epidemiology."[6]

Meta-Analysis

A meta-analysis consists of a critical evaluation of research studies that statistically combines the results of comparable studies or clinical trials on a specific topic. Unlike review articles, which can be qualitative or narrative in form, a meta-analysis is a statistical tool that can be used to quantitatively synthesize the findings of different studies.

Although a standardized strategy for conducting a meta-analysis has not been accepted, researchers agree on the following procedures:

- Study protocol. The analysis must begin with a protocol that states the purpose, methodology, and criteria for selection of studies.
- Selection of studies. Primary source papers of empirically based studies, usually experimental studies, must be used.
- Statistical analysis. Statistical procedures for combining the results of these studies must be rigorously followed.

There is continuing disagreement about other issues, including the criteria for including and excluding primary studies, whether or not the papers have to have been published, and whether the data to be analyzed have to be at the study or the individual subject level.[7]

Just as there are criteria for a well-done research study and others for evaluating the quality of a review article, there are also guidelines for a well-done meta-analysis. One set of guidelines was published as a series of articles in the *British Medical Journal* in 1997 and 1998; additional articles are expected to be published in the future.[8-13]

Practice Guidelines

Clinical practice guidelines were defined in 1992 by the Institute of Medicine, as "systematically developed statements to assist practitioner and patient decisions about appropriate health care for specific clinical circumstances."[14] Further information is available at http://www.nap.edu/readingroom/records/0309045894.htm/. See also the paper by Lohr.[15] Some practice guidelines are for community interventions such as immunization rather than for individual patients. For example, see the 1994 paper by Gyorkos, "An approach to the development of practice guidelines for community health interventions."[16]

Cochrane Library

The Cochrane Library is an electronic library of systematic reviews of health-related research findings. A standard protocol is used for all Cochrane reviews, as described in the Cochrane Collaboration Handbook,[17] which can be found on the Cochrane web site at http://www.wepublish.com/cochranehandbook/default.htm/.

The Cochrane reviews, first released in April 1996, are updated on a quarterly basis and are available by subscription on CD-ROM or via the Internet. Many university libraries have a subscription to the CD-ROM and make the information available free of charge to their patrons. Check with the reference librarian. A considerable amount of information is also available on the Internet. For example, see http://www.cochrane.org/.

Currently, the Cochrane Library consists of the following 4 databases.

1. **Cochrane Database of Systematic Reviews (CDSR).** CDSR is a collection of systematic reviews of the effects of experimental studies of health care. Each review is prepared by one of the voluntary Cochrane Collaborative Review Groups using pre-approved protocols for research synthesis as specified in the Cochrane Review Methodology Database. The reviews are updated and amended as new evidence becomes available. The

CDSR is the primary output of the collaborative. Examples of some of the reviews include the following, as described by the Canadian members of the Cochrane Collaborative based at McMaster University:

- how stroke can be prevented and treated,
- which drugs are effective in the treatment of malaria, tuberculosis, and other infectious diseases, and
- which strategies are effective in preventing brain and spinal cord injuries and their consequences.

The website of the McMaster group is http://hiru.mcmaster.ca/cochrane/cochrane/general.htm/.

2. **Database of Abstracts of Reviews of Effectiveness (DARE).** This contains abstracts of other systematic reviews based on explicit criteria, abstracts from health technology agencies from around the world, and abstracts of reviews prior to 1995 by members of the American College of Physicians' Journal Club. DARE is maintained by National Health Service's Centre for Reviews and Dissemination in York, England.

3. **Cochrane Controlled Trials Register.** This is a bibliographic database of randomized clinical trials or experimental studies of health care interventions that include trials described in conference proceedings and other sources not usually available in peer-reviewed journals.

4. **Cochrane Review Methodology Database.** This includes publications in journals and books about the science of reviewing research. Also included in this database is a handbook of how to conduct a systematic review and a glossary of terms. The database also describes how to contact the Cochrane Library and information about Collaborative Review Groups.

The Cochrane Library is rapidly evolving and may eventually become the primary international source of information about the effectiveness of health care interventions. This is an important resource for anyone interested in the synthesis of findings about health care interventions across multiple research studies.

Using Tertiary Source Materials

In reading a review article, results of a meta-analysis, practice guidelines, or material from the Cochrane Library, pay special attention to the list of papers in the references section. These references may be useful as you search for primary source articles.

Given the systematic effort and expertise that go into creating many of these tertiary source materials, you may now be wondering why you should do your own review of the literature. Why not simply use the excellent output of others on the topic of your choice? The answer is threefold:

- The purpose of your review of the literature may not be exactly what has been included in these tertiary source materials.
- A secondary or tertiary source document will inevitably contain a bias that you may or may not recognize. So far as that goes, *your* review of the primary source materials will also contain a bias. The advantage of doing your own review is that of experience—you know what the researchers said they did and how you interpreted their methods and results. You do not have that level of understanding if you read someone else's synthesis or review of the same documents.
- Finally, you will not truly own the literature without examining the actual, primary source documents yourself. This is especially important for future research. On the other hand, if your goal is to gain a better understanding about what interventions or treatments are effective, then using one or more of the tertiary source documents may be the most efficient strategy.

Each of the 4 examples of tertiary source information has strengths and weaknesses. Reviews can vary in thoroughness and quality. There are no standards for review articles, as has been pointed out by others in the field. The same concern applies to a meta-analysis. A statistical methodology does not automatically confer objectivity. How the studies were selected initially, the quality of those original studies, and the appropriateness of the meta-analytic techniques are important considerations. Practice guidelines were developed for practitioners and the quality of the research and ways in which the studies were combined to arrive at the guidelines may vary. Finally, the emphasis in the systematic reviews by the Cochrane Collaborative is on randomized trials. There is a vast amount of useful information from research studies that do not use that particular methodological design, and those studies are not emphasized in the Cochrane Library. In summary, you should seriously consider using tertiary source documents, but only as an adjunct to primary and secondary source materials.

The Internet and World Wide Web: Beware of Readily Available Resources

The Internet and the World Wide Web (www), which is currently the most popular system for accessing the Internet, offer expanding opportunities for the reviewer of the literature. One of the first places to explore is the U.S. National Library of Medicine (NLM) at http://www.nlm.gov/. The NLM, which is part of the National Institutes of Health (NIH), has developed and maintains MEDLINE and other health-related databases. The web site of the National Institutes of Health is http://www.nih.gov/. Both of these sites—the National Library of Medicine and the National Institutes of Health—can also be found by typing in these names in the search fields of most search engines.

Other sites to explore include professional associations that publish journals, for example, the American Medical Association which publishes the *Journal of the American Medical Association (JAMA)* or the American Sociological Society which publishes the *Journal of Health and Social Behavior*. Alternatively, you could search for the names of specific journals, such as the *American Journal of Public Health* or *Science*. Appendix A includes a list of some of the more well-known scientific associations and their web sites.

Access to MEDLINE is available without charge on the Internet at http://www.nlm.nih.gov/databases/freemedl.html/. A list of on-line journals that has been compiled by the National Library of Medicine is available at http://www.ncbi.nlm.nih.gov/PubMed/fulltext.html/.

The credibility of electronic sources can vary, depending on who or what organization has produced the information. Some general sources on the Internet that may be helpful in evaluating electronic sources include the following:

- Thinking critically about World Wide Web resources, by Ester Grassian, available at http://www.library.ucla.edu/libraries/college/instruct/critical.htm/
- Evaluating World Wide Web information, by Purdue University, available at http://thorplus.lib.purdue.edu/research/classes/gs175/3gs175/evaluation.html/
- Teaching students to think critically about Internet resources, available at http://weber.u.washington.edu/~lbr560/NETEVAL/index.html/
- Bibliography on evaluating Internet resources, available at http://refserver.lib.vt.edu/libinst/critTHINK.HTM/

Computer Retrieval of Information on Scientific Projects (CRISP)

In reviewing the literature, it is sometimes important to know about studies that are in progress, even if the results are not yet available. For example, if you are thinking about applying for a grant proposal, it is important to find out if a similar study has already been funded. Alternatively, you might have a pressing clinical or patient-related problem for which there is little or no information in the literature, and you need to find out who in the country is doing research on that issue. Finally, you may want to identify researchers who have not yet published in an area, but who might be presenting results at upcoming scientific meetings. By identifying current research projects, you could follow them in future literature or contact the researchers directly about their plans for publication of results.

Although a list of all research studies ever conducted or even those currently in progress does not exist, you can identify many of the research projects funded by the federal government by examining the Computer Retrieval of Information on Scientific Projects (CRISP). CRISP is a searchable database of federally funded biomedical research projects conducted at universities, hospitals, and other research institutions. Projects that have been completed as well as those currently in progress are included in the CRISP database.

CRISP is maintained by the National Institutes of Health and includes studies funded by NIH, Substance Abuse and Mental Health Services Administration (SAMSHA), Health Resources and Services Administration (HRSA), Food and Drug Administration (FDA), Centers for Disease Control and Prevention (CDCP), Agency for Health Care Policy Research (AHCPR), and Office of Assistant Secretary of Health (OASH).

CRISP is available on the Internet at either of the following URLs: http://www-commons.dcrt.nih.gov:80/index.html/, then choose CRISP on the list on the left. An alternative URL is http://eos12.dcrt.nih.gov:8002/crisp_pilot/owa/crisp.main/. If neither of these URLs is available in the future, access the home page of the National Institutes of Health and search for CRISP.

In general, running a CRISP search is one of the first steps to take in thinking about developing a grant proposal to be submitted to the NIH or one of the other nationally competitive funding organizations. This is also a quick way to learn about developments in the field before they become available in the research literature.

There are other searchable databases of research grants and clinical trials in specific disciplines. Information about many of these databases can be found at the Internet Grateful Med web site, http://igm.nlm.nih.gov/, maintained by the NLM. An example of one of the NLM databases is HSRProj, which contains descriptions of research in progress funded by federal and private grants and contracts for use by policy makers, managers, clinicians, and other decision makers. It provides access to information about health services research in progress before results are available in a published form. The HSRProj website is http://www.nlm.nih.gov/pubs/factsheets/online. databases.html#hsrproj/.

Citation Index: A Useful Tool Once You Know What You Want

Once you are well into the process of locating specific journals and doing an initial reading of primary source materials, determine whether there are some individuals who consistently have been associated with the topic of interest. For example, are there key scientists who were the first to do this kind of research or authors whose seminal papers are almost always cited by others in their publications? If so, consider using the *Science Citation Index* (or its social sciences counterpart, the *Social Science Citation Index*) to identify other scientific publications in which the researchers list the papers by the key authors. Citation indexes are available in print (and often in electronic) form in most research libraries; the reference librarian will be able to help you locate and use such indexes.

In one sense, these citation indexes work backwards. For example, suppose that 2 fictitious researchers, Smith and Jones, published the first major study of quality of life of women with breast cancer in 1956 in the (fictitious) *Journal of American Health*, and their research was so important that most other researchers in the future cited that original paper. Now, years later, you want to identify all studies on this topic that have been reported since the Smith and Jones 1956 paper. Using the *Science Citation Index*, you look up Smith and Jones, and among their many publications, you locate the 1956 *Journal of American Health* article. Listed under that article will be a list of other studies, from 1956 to the present, that included the Smith and Jones article in the reference lists of their papers. In other words, the Smith and Jones 1956 paper was cited by these other authors. Such a list could be invaluable in a review of the literature because it quickly and efficiently gives you a list of potentially related articles that you can then examine and consider including in your review of the literature.

TIPS ON SEARCHING FOR SOURCE DOCUMENTS

Snowballing Technique: Developing Ownership of the Literature

Use what is known as the snowball technique to find more references. A snowball gathers snow as it rolls down the hill, and by the same token, your goal should be to use references in the papers or books you have read to gather more references. Even if a particular article in a journal is not relevant to the topic under review, some of the references might be. Build a list of references until you begin to see the same references over and over again. In fact, an author's failure to cite an important article in a current publication might suggest that this author did not fully read the literature, which might also make you question the quality of the study. You will know that you are beginning to own the literature when you read a few sentences about a study cited by an author and you immediately think to yourself, "Oh yes, that was the study by Smith and Jones in which they found that . . ." even before you see the reference to Smith and Jones at the end of the description.

Timeliness of the Science: A Comparison of Sources

One consideration in reviewing the literature might be whether or not to include the most recent findings on a topic. Unfortunately, by the time a scientific paper is published in a peer-reviewed journal, the results are already out of date in some fields. Probably the most current knowledge about a topic can be found in papers presented at scientific meetings— but this applies only to the day or week they are presented. The disadvantage of presentations at scientific meetings is that they usually have not been subjected to the rigorous review process required of papers published in peer-reviewed journals. Materials made available on the Internet might also be very recent, but they are probably even more suspect if they have not gone through the peer-review process. The exception might be on-line, full-text papers in peer-reviewed journals available on the Internet. Examples of on-line journals are included in Appendix A. In general, the most recent published studies are papers in scientific journals, followed by those described in the annual reviews, followed lastly by books.

If you restrict the review to scientific, peer-reviewed, hard copy, published journals, then how recent is recent? The time from completion of a study (or the end of the study period, since it is not always clear when the study actually ended) to publication varies from study to study and field to field. Try to get a sense of a relative definition of recentness for papers in some journals by noting when the papers were submitted or accepted and when they were published. You will need to delve further, however, to discover how much time elapsed between completion of the study and when the paper was submitted or accepted.

Take for example all of the patient-related articles that were original contributions published in the 4 June 1998 issue of the *Journal of the American Medical Association*. There were 14 such articles, summarized in Exhibit 3-4, of which 2 did not provide information about when the data were collected or the study period ended. As shown in the last column of Exhibit 3-4, the range of time elapsed between the end of the data collection period (or end of study) and the publication of these 12 papers was 15 to 89 months. Thus, the information in the (then) latest issue of one of the foremost clinical journals in the world was published 3.67 years, on the average, after the data were collected.

Research takes time, and good research often takes a lot of time. In thinking about the number of months or years elapsed between the end of study and publication of results, perhaps the most important issue to consider is how recent the findings have to be for the information to be meaningful to health providers and of benefit to their patients.

Exhibit 3-4 Time Elapsed between End of Study and Publication of Final Results in the June 1998 Issue of the *Journal of the American Medical Association (JAMA)*

Study Description	Date of Publication in JAMA	End of Study Period or Completion of Data Collection*	Number of Months Elapsed: End of Study to Publication
Socioeconomic Factors, Health Behaviors, and Mortality[18]	6/3/98	3/1/94	50
Perceived Prognosis and Treatment Preference[19]	6/3/98	1/1/94	52
Cigarette Smoking and Hearing Loss[20]	6/3/98	1995	29
Depressive Symptoms and Physical Decline[21]	6/3/98	1992	65
Death After Hospital Discharge[22]	6/3/98	1994	41
Low Back Pain in Industry[23]	6/10/98	N/A	N/A
Unintentional Cocaine Overdose[24]	6/10/98	12/31/95	29
Culture, Race, and Breast Cancer Stage[25]	6/10/98	N/A	N/A
Pain Management in Elderly Patients With Cancer[26]	6/17/98	1995	17

continues

Exhibit 3-4 continued

Study Description	Date of Publication in JAMA	End of Study Period or Completion of Data Collection*	Number of Months Elapsed: End of Study to Publication
HIV Incidence Among Young Adults[27]	6/17/98	1993	53
Risk Factors in Ischemic Heart Disease[28]	6/24/98	1990	89
Zinc Gluconate Lozenges for the Common Cold[29]	6/24/98	3/97	15
Adjusting Cesarean Delivery Rates[30]	6/24/98	6/95	36
Gastrostomies in Medicare Beneficiaries[31]	6/24/98	12/93	53

*When only the year of data collection was reported, the ending date was set to December of that year, unless otherwise noted in the paper. N/A = Not Available

Caroline's Quest: Managing the Search

For her thesis research, Caroline was interested in studying the characteristics of teenage girls who smoke. She was especially interested in exploring whether or not there was a link between smoking and depression. In order to design her study, Caroline first needed to know what the research literature had shown about both the prevalence of smoking in that age and gender group and what kinds of characteristics had been studied thus far. She knew from previous reading that race or ethnic origin, socioeconomic status, and rural/urban location were probably important factors, but she wasn't sure what other kinds of characteristics had been studied.

After talking with Professor Dickerson, Caroline decided to begin by briefly reading pertinent chapters in a few reference books, then concentrating her search for primary source documents by looking in MEDLINE, and next examining some tertiary source documents beginning with the Cochrane Library.

At the library, Caroline skimmed the material on the topic of smoking and teenagers in the reference books and made some notes about these reference materials under Key Sources in the Paper Trail section of her Lit Review Book, as shown in Exhibit 3-5.

Prior to doing a MEDLINE search, Caroline listed some key words and set some initial restrictions for the search. She decided to focus only on American teenagers, with an age range of 13–18 years, if possible. She also wanted to limit

---

Exhibit 3-5 Key Sources Page in the Paper Trail Section of Caroline's Lit Review Book

Preventing tobacco use among young people: a report of the Surgeon General: at a glance. 1994. National Center for Chronic Disease Prevention and Health Program.

her MEDLINE search to the most recent 10 years. Under Professor Dickerson's guidance, she was aware that the definitions and terms for her search could be modified as she learned more about her topic.

Caroline wrote this information down in the Notes subsection in her Paper Trail section in order to have a record of her decisions about the MEDLINE search. Her notes are shown in Exhibit 3-6.

Next she turned to the page titled, Key Words, in the Paper Trail section and described the purpose of her literature review and some of the key words that she would use initially. Exhibit 3-7 is a record of what she wrote.

Caroline was able to access a variety of electronic bibliographic databases, such as MEDLINE, from the computer in her office, rather than go to the library. She

---

Exhibit 3-6 Notes Page in the Paper Trail Section of Caroline's Lit Review Book

---

Subject characteristics
- Teenage—ages 13–18 years
- Smoking—use cigarette smoking only

Prevalence—be sure to get prevalence (rate of people currently smoking divided by total number at risk for smoking). May need to do this on a year-by-year basis. Wonder if I can get this for the whole age period? May want to set up a graph showing prevalence by year for each age.

Limit search to the following:
- The most recent 10 years, at least initially
- Focus only on American teenagers because they might differ from other cultures
- Separate different ethnic groups within the U.S., e.g., Caucasian, African-American, Asian, American Indian—there may be different characteristics associated with smoking within each ethnic group
- Limit search to English language journals only
- Check review articles, then go to the actual studies

Exhibit 3-7 Key Words Page in the Paper Trail Section of Caroline's Lit Review Book

> **Purpose**
> What are the characteristics of teenage girls who smoke during the period 1985 to the present in the U.S.?
> **Key Words**
>   smoking
>   cigarettes
>   teenage girls
>   prevalence of smoking among teenage girls

also had 2 options for accessing the MEDLINE database. One was through PubMed, which was free via the Internet, and the other was through the OVID system, which was available through the biomedical library she used, although Professor Dickerson had told her that not all university libraries provide OVID free of charge to its users. Each had slightly different capabilities, although both provided a gateway to MEDLINE. She decided to use the PubMed system initially.

Caroline logged onto the Internet and, prior to going to the PubMed web site, she checked the home page of the National Library of Medicine, www.nlm.nih.gov/, to see if there were any new features that had become available. Then she went directly to the PubMed site, www.ncbi.nlm.nih.gov/PubMed/, to begin her MEDLINE search. The PubMed screen she went to first is shown in Figure 3-1.

Using the PubMed search capability, Caroline began her search with the key word phrase, "smoking/epidemiology," then restricted the search by the age and nationality criteria she had previously established. A copy of Caroline's first query, which retrieved 4,631 documents, is shown in Figure 3-2.

Caroline applied the search restrictions she had decided on earlier and recorded the results in the Notes subsection of her Paper Trail. Her search resulted in 235 references, as shown in Exhibit 3-8.

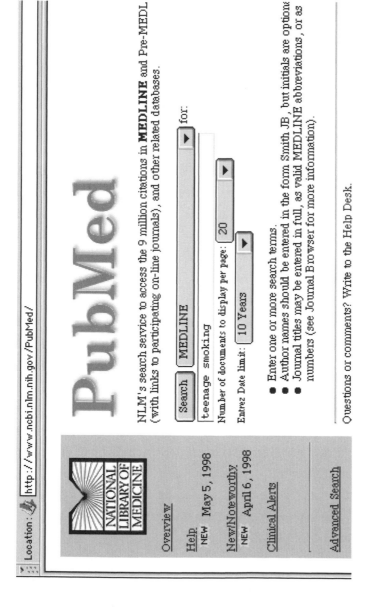

Figure 3-1 PubMed Web Site That Caroline Accessed To Use MEDLINE. *Source:* Copyright Netscape Communications Corporation, 1998. All Rights Reserved. Netscape, Netscape Navigator, and the Netscape logo are registered trademarks of Netscape in the United States and other countries.

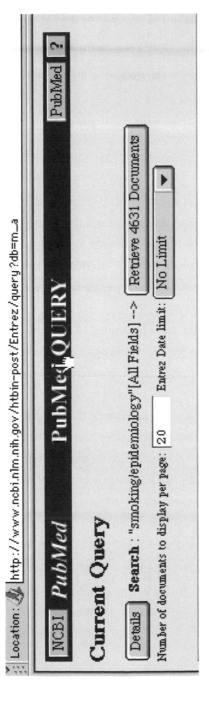

Figure 3-2 Results of Caroline's Initial Query of the MEDLINE Database Using "smoking/epidemiology" as the Key Word Phrase. *Source:* Copyright Netscape Communications Corporation, 1998. All Rights Reserved. Netscape, Netscape Navigator, and the Netscape logo are registered trademarks of Netscape in the United States and other countries.

Exhibit 3-8 Notes Page in the Paper Trail Section of Caroline's Lit Review Book

Key words	Number of references
smoking/	
epidemiology	4,631
English language	3,954
human subjects	3,941
adolescents	235

Next, Caroline scanned the titles and abstracts of each of the 235 citations until she found a title relating to adolescents and smoking: the 1996 Altman, et al. citation shown in Figure 3-3.

She examined the abstract, shown in Figure 3-4. Then she returned to the citations list and clicked on See Related Articles to find additional studies on the same topics.

Unfortunately, the full text of the paper by Altman, et al., was not available online, which meant that in order to read the entire paper, she had to get a hard copy from the journal at the library. She repeated this procedure with the rest of the 235 citations until she had approximately 15 abstracts to examine in greater depth.

Caroline also explored some of the other electronic bibliographic databases such as CancerLit and Current Contents. Much of what she had found in MEDLINE was included in those 2 databases, although there were a few differences. Then she went to the biomedical library and made a photocopy of each of the papers she had chosen to consider in her literature review.

Later, Caroline returned to the Internet to look for reviews completed by members of the Cochrane Collaboration. She reasoned that these tertiary source materials might provide additional references of original research studies. She logged onto the Cochrane Collaboration home page at http://hiru.mcmaster.ca/cochrane/cochrane/general.htm/ which is shown in Figure 3-5.

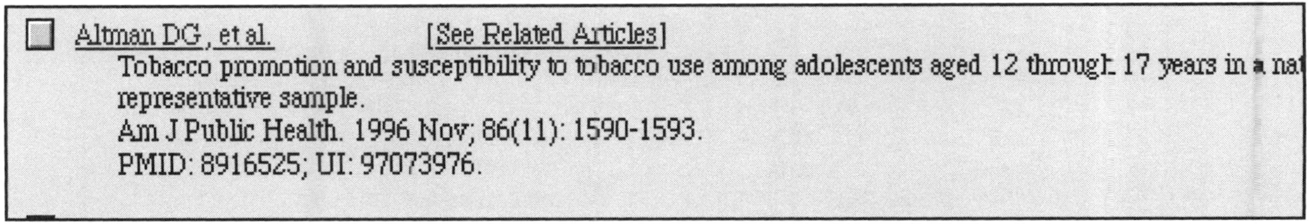

Altman DG, et al.   [See Related Articles]
   Tobacco promotion and susceptibility to tobacco use among adolescents aged 12 through 17 years in a nat
   representative sample.
   Am J Public Health. 1996 Nov; 86(11): 1590-1593.
   PMID: 8916525; UI: 97073976.

Figure 3-3 Example of Reference from MEDLINE. *Source:* Copyright Netscape Communications Corporation, 1998. All Rights Reserved. Netscape, Netscape Navigator and the Netscape logo are registered trademarks of Netscape in the United States and other countries.

Am J Public Health 1996 Nov;86(11):1590-1593

Tobacco promotion and susceptibility to tobacco use among adolescents aged 12 through 17 years in a nationally representative sample.

Altman DG, Levine DW, Coeytaux R, Slade J, Jaffe R

Bowman Gray School of Medicine, Department of Public Health Sciences, Winston-Salem, NC 27157-1063, USA.

OBJECTIVES: The purpose of this study was to examine whether youth participation in tobacco promotion campaigns is associated with susceptibility to tobacco use. METHODS: Data were collected from telephone interviews of a national random sample of 1047 adolescents 12 to 17 years of age. RESULTS: A proportional odds model was used to estimate the effects of age, gender, presence of a tobacco user in the household, awareness of tobacco promotions, knowledge of a young adult or adolescent friend owning a promotional item, participation in tobacco promotions, and receipt of free tobacco samples or direct mail from tobacco companies on susceptibility to tobacco use. All of the covariates, except for receiving direct mailings and knowing a young adult friend who owned a promotional item, were significantly associated with susceptibility.

Figure 3-4 Abstract Caroline Chose To Examine. *Source:* Adapted from the National Library of Medicine. Adapted with permission from D.G. Altman, et al., Tobacco Promotion and Susceptibility to Tobacco Use Among Adolescents Aged 12 Through 17 Years in a Nationally Representative Sample. *American Journal of Public Health*, Vol. 86, No. 11, pp. 1590–1593, © 1996, American Public Health Association.

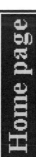

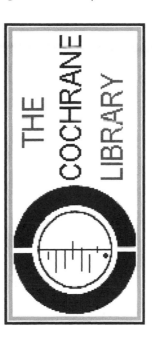

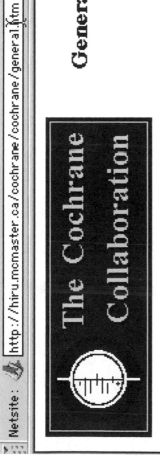

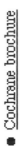

Netsite: http://hiru.mcmaster.ca/cochrane/cochrane/general.htm

General Information

THE COCHRANE LIBRARY

The Cochrane Collaboration

● Cochrane brochure
● Cochrane leaflet
● Cochrane documents
● Cochrane Library and Review Abstracts
● Cochrane Groups and Centres
● Annual International Colloquia
● Newsletters
● Workshops and Training

Home page

Figure 3-5 Cochrane Collaboration Home Page that Caroline Accessed. *Source:* Courtesy of Cochrane Collaboration, Baltimore, Maryland. Copyright Netscape Communications Corporation, 1998. All Rights Reserved. Netscape, Netscape Navigator, and the Netscape logo are registered trademarks of Netscape in the United States and other countries.

She clicked the Review Abstracts on the Home Page in order to determine if any Cochrane Reviews had been completed for smoking. She found a list of all reviews to date at the next site under Collaborative Review Groups, shown at the bottom of the screen in Figure 3-6.

One of these groups included the Tobacco Addiction Group. She went to that site and found a list of 10 reviews and 3 protocols, as shown in Figure 3-7.

Although none of the reviews was exactly in the area of her interest, the third protocol on mass media interventions looked like it might have some relevance to her topic.

Professor Dickinson had told her that the protocols in the Cochrane Library were reviews in progress, so she clicked on the third protocol to find out who was doing it and whether there was any further information. She printed out the names of the protocol team and made a note to ask Professor Dickerson about the protocol at their next meeting. She made a bookmark of the web site in order to check it out at a later date.

Caroline decided to examine some other tertiary sources. She was particularly interested in looking in the *Annual Review of Public Health* to see if there was an article on her topic. She reasoned that a current review would give her a list of up-to-date references of original studies that would be useful to examine. She went first to the *Annual Reviews* web site, http://www.annualreviews.org/, and then to the site for the *Annual Review of Public Health*. She did not find any review articles that were specific to her topic; therefore she decided to concentrate on reading the 15 papers she had photocopied to decide which of those should be included in her review. Then she would use the references from those papers to help her identify additional studies. Perhaps later she would consider using the *Science Citation Index*.

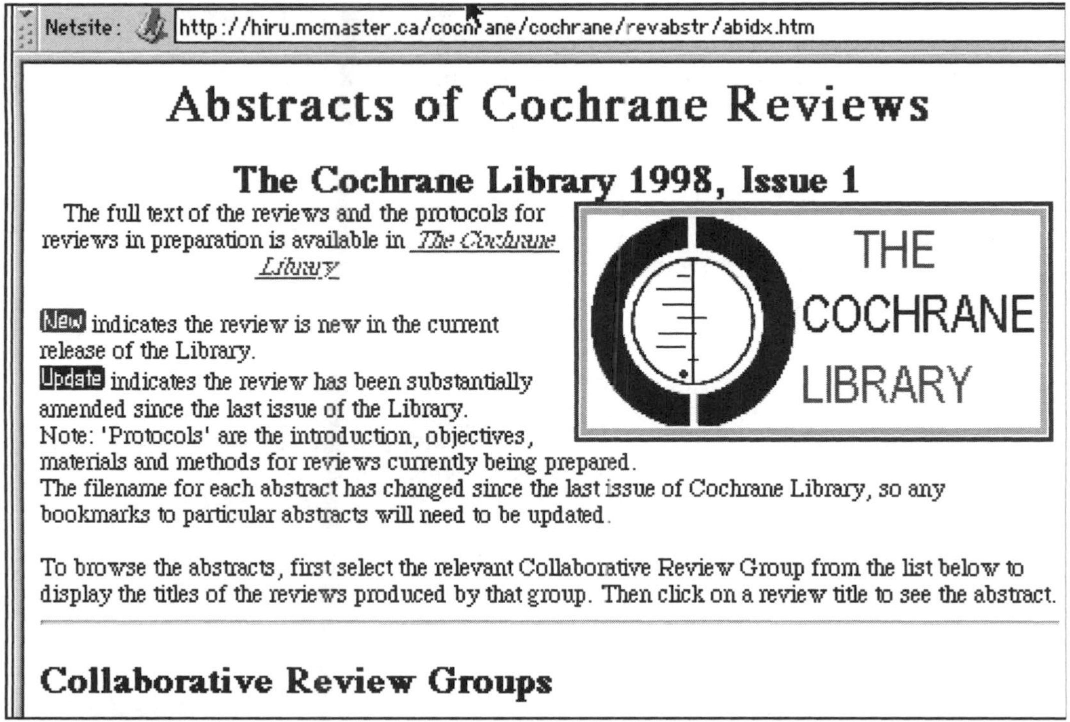

Figure 3-6 Abstracts of Cochrane Reviews. Courtesy of Cochrane Collaboration, Baltimore, Maryland. Copyright Netscape Communications Corporation, 1998. All Rights Reserved. Netscape, Netscape Navigator, and the Netscape logo are registered trademarks of Netscape in the United States and other countries.

Netsite: http://hiru.mcmaster.ca/cochrane/cochrane/revabstr/abidx6.htm#G16@

TOBACCO ADDICTION GROUP

Reviews

- Acupuncture in smoking cessation
- Anxiolytics and antidepressants in smoking cessation
- Clonidine for smoking cessation
- Lobeline for smoking cessation
- Mecamylamine (a nicotine antagonist) for smoking cessation
- Nicotine replacement therapy for smoking cessation
- Physician advice for smoking cessation
- Silver acetate for smoking cessation
- The effect of aversive smoking on smoking cessation
- Training health professionals to provide smoking cessation interventions

Protocols

- Group behaviour therapy programmes for smoking cessation
- Hypnotherapy for smoking cessation
- Mass media interventions for preventing smoking among young people

Figure 3-7 Tobacco Addiction Group Accessed by Caroline. Courtesy of Cochrane Collaboration, Baltimore, Maryland. Copyright Netscape Communications Corporation, 1998. All Rights Reserved. Netscape, Netscape Navigator, and the Netscape logo are registered trademarks of Netscape in the United States and other countries.

REFERENCES

1. Poikolainen K. Alcohol and mortality: A review. *J Clin Epidemiol.* 1995;48:455–456.
2. Hunt DL, McKibbon KA. Locating and appraising systematic reviews. *Annals of Internal Medicine.* 1997;126:532–538.
3. Weed DL. Methodologic guidelines for review papers. *Journal of the National Cancer Institute.* 1997;89:6–7.
4. Oxman AD, Guyatt GH, Cook DJ, Jaeschke R, Heddle N, Keller J. An index of scientific quality for health reports in the lay press. *Journal of Clinical Epidemiology.* 1993;46:987–1001.
5. Oxman AD. Checklists for review articles. *BMJ.* 1994;309:648–651.
6. Breslow RA, Ross SA, Weed DL. Quality of reviews in epidemiology. *American Journal of Public Health.* 1998;88:475–477.
7. Fagard RH, Staessen JA, Thijs L. Advantages and disadvantages of the meta-analysis approach. *Journal of Hypertension—Supplement.* 1996;14: S9–12; discussion S13.
8. Egger M, Smith GD. Meta-analysis. Potentials and promise. *BMJ.* 1997;315:1371–1374.
9. Egger M, Smith GD, Phillips AN. Meta-analysis: principles and procedures. *BMJ.* 1997;315:1533–1537.
10. Davey Smith G, Egger M, Phillips AN. Meta-analysis. Beyond the grand mean? *BMJ.* 1997;315:1610–1614.
11. Egger M, Smith GD. Bias in location and selection of studies. *BMJ.* 1998;316:61–66.
12. Egger M, Schneider M, Smith GD. Meta-analysis—Spurious Precision—Meta-analysis of observational studies. *BMJ.* 1998;316:140–144.
13. Davey Smith G, Egger M. Meta-analysis. Unresolved issues and future developments. *BMJ.* 1998;316:221–225.
14. Field MJ, Lohr KN. *Guidelines for Clinical Practice: From Development to Use.* Washington DC: Committee on Clinical Practice Guidelines, Division of Health Care Services, Institute of Medicine; 1992.
15. Lohr KN. Guidelines for clinical practice: What they are and why they count. *Journal of Law, Medicine & Ethics.* 1995;23:49–56.
16. Gyorkos TW, Tannenbaum TN, Abrahamowicz M, et al. An approach to the development of practice guidelines for community health interventions. *Canadian Journal of Public Health.* 1994;85:S8–13.
17. Mulrow CD, Oxman AD. Cochrane Collaboration Handbook [updated September 1997]. In: The Cochrane Library [database on disk and CDROM]. In: Mulrow CD, Oxman AD, eds. *The Cochrane Collaboration.* Oxford: Update Software; 1997.

18. Lantz PM, House JS, Lepkowski JM, Williams DR, Mero RP, Chen J. Socioeconomic factors, health behaviors, and mortality: Results from a nationally representative prospective study of US adults. *JAMA.* 1998; 279:1703–1708.

19. Weeks JC, Cook EF, O'Day SJ, et al. Relationship between cancer patients' predictions of prognosis and their treatment preferences. *JAMA.* 1998;279:1709–1714.

20. Cruickshanks KJ, Klein R, Klein BE, Wiley TL, Nordahl DM, Tweed TS. Cigarette smoking and hearing loss: The epidemiology of hearing loss study. *JAMA.* 1998;279:1715–1726.

21. Penninx BWJH, Guralnik JM, Ferrucci L, Simonsick EM, Deeg DJH, Wallace RB. Depressive symptoms and physical decline in community-dwelling older persons. *JAMA.* 1998;279:1720–1726.

22. Mullins RJ, Mann NC, Hedges JR, et al. Adequacy of hospital discharge status as a measure of outcome among injured patients. *JAMA.* 1998;279:1227–1231.

23. van Poppel NMN, Koes BW, van der Ploeg T, Smid T, Bouter LM. Lumbar supports and education for the prevention of low back pain in industry: A randomized controlled trial. *JAMA.* 1998;279:1789–1794.

24. Marzuk PM, Tardiff K, Leon AC, et al. Ambient temperature and mortality from unintentional cocaine overdose. *JAMA.* 1998;279:1795–1800.

25. Lannin DR, Mathews HF, Mitchell J, Swanson MS, Swanson FH, Edwards MS. Influence of socioeconomic and cultural factors on racial differences in late-stage presentation of breast cancer. *JAMA.* 1998;279:1801–1807.

26. Bernabei R, Gambassi G, Lapane K, et al. Management of pain in elderly patients with cancer. *JAMA.* 1998;279:1877–1882.

27. Rosenberg PS, Biggar RJ. Trends in HIV incidence among young adults in the United States. *JAMA.* 1998;279:1894–1899.

28. Lamarche B, Tchernof A, Mauriege P, et al. Fasting insulin and apolipoprotein B levels and low-density lipoprotein particle size as risk factors for ischemic heart disease. *JAMA.* 1998;279:1955–1961.

29. Macknin ML, Piedmonte M, Calendine C, Janosky J, Wald E. Zinc gluconate lozenges for treating the common cold in children: A randomized controlled trial. *JAMA.* 1998;279:1962–1967.

30. Aron DC, Harper DL, Shepardson LB, Rosenthal GE. Impact of risk-adjusting cesarean delivery rates when reporting hospital performance. *JAMA.* 1998;279:1968–1972.

31. Grant MD, Rudberg MA, Brody JA. Gastrostomy placement and mortality among hospitalized medicare beneficiaries. *JAMA.* 1998;279: 1973–1976.

Documents Section: How To Select and Organize Documents for Review

This chapter is about how to select, organize, and keep track of all the documents you use in a review of the literature. It includes the following five sections:

- ☑ How To Select the Right Documents for Your Review
- ☑ What Is a Documents Section?
- ☑ How To Organize a Documents Section
- ☑ How To Remember Where You Put the Documents
- ☑ Caroline's Quest: Assembling a Documents Section

HOW TO SELECT THE RIGHT
DOCUMENTS FOR YOUR REVIEW

Selecting documents to include as possible candidates for your literature review is your next task. Reviewing the abstract, skimming the document, and photocopying the document are the 3 steps of the Matrix Method process for selecting documents.

Review the Abstract

If the document is an original research article, then quickly read the abstract to see if it is relevant to your topic. This strategy is most efficient if the abstract is available on-line in a database such as MEDLINE. Unfortunately, not all papers have an abstract, nor do the electronic bibliographic databases provide abstracts for some kinds of documents. For example, editorials usually do not include an abstract, yet such a document may include an important issue or a significant reference. Furthermore, some journals do not require an abstract for any of the papers. For documents with those limitations, go to the actual journal or source to determine if they need to be considered for your review.

Skim the Document

If either the title of the article or the abstract appears to be relevant to your topic or the study has been mentioned in a secondary or tertiary source document, the next step is to briefly examine the original article. You will be fortunate if you can find the article as a full-text, on-line document—in other words, reprinted in its entirety in electronic form. Certainly it is a lot easier to sit at your desk and click to a web site to examine a paper than it is to get up and go to the library. Usually, you will not be so fortunate, at least not at this point in time. Nor should you even consider limiting your search to only those articles reproduced in electronic form. There are not enough of them, and the sample of such journals is likely to be biased.

Once the paper is in hand, skim it briefly to determine whether or not it is relevant to your topic. Look not only at the abstract, but also the entire article, including the authors' statement of the purpose, the methods section, and the results. Consider the possibility that while the topic of a paper may be too specific for your review, the methods or the conclusions may have some relevance to a discussion in your final synthesis of the literature. In that case, make a copy of the article.

This article selection process alone is not sufficient for a review of the literature. This is just the beginning. This stage involves only making a decision about whether or not to keep a copy of the document for possible inclusion in your review.

Photocopy the Document

Depending on your budget, make a copy of relevant articles. If financial resources are tight, organize the documents on a continuum from clearly essential to maybe relevant to remotely interesting and photocopy from the top down until you run out of money. This means, however, that you may have to return to the library at an inconvenient time to re-examine one or more of the maybe relevant articles.

Once you have selected a set of source documents, the next step is to use them to create the Documents section of your Lit Review Book.

WHAT IS A DOCUMENTS SECTION?

The Documents section of a Lit Review Book consists of 1 copy of each of the papers or source documents assembled for the literature review. In the years before photocopy machines were routinely available, you would have written to the author and asked for a reprint of the paper. Then, as now, most scientific journals offered authors these reprints free or at cost. The practice of requesting a reprint is not as common now as in the past because most journals are available in major research libraries, through interlibrary loan, or more recently as full-text files on the Internet, and users can simply make a copy themselves. The term *reprint* is still with us, however, and occasionally you hear a collection of journal articles assembled for a review of the literature referred to as a "reprint file." Thus the Documents section is the same as a reprints file.

Think of the Documents section as your hard-copy database. This will be an incomplete database, however, since some documents are too large (books, for example), unavailable (the library doesn't carry the journal), or restricted (such as proprietary materials owned by a private company). Maintain a list of all source documents that are important for your review, whether or not a copy is available. Often, books can be obtained through interlibrary loan, and a copy of an article in an unavailable journal might be requested through the same source or from the author. Proprietary materials present another problem that may not be surmounted, but listing those that appear to be relevant in an appendix in your synthesis will indicate the thoroughness of your search.

Advantages of a Documents Section

The advantage of keeping a Documents section is being able to find your copy of a document when you need it. Even experienced researchers sometimes have trouble locating copies of reprints. Occasionally, these seasoned veterans take the precaution of making multiple copies and spreading them around in several files in order to increase the likelihood of finding a copy when they need it. A Documents section in a Lit Review Book solves that problem by providing a central resource for all reprints or photocopies of research articles.

HOW TO ORGANIZE A DOCUMENTS SECTION

Just having a copy of a source document in the Documents section does not guarantee that you will be able to find it efficiently the next time you need it. To bring order to the Documents section organize the materials by year of publication.

Using index tabs, divide the Documents section by year, with the earliest year at the beginning and the most recent year at the end. In other words, file your documents chronologically from earliest to latest. As you accumulate source documents, write the year of publication at the top right-hand corner of each article and use it as the sorting key. Any further organization of the articles in the Documents section such as alphabetizing or grouping together by content area within a year, probably is not necessary.

The goal of this chronological sequence is twofold: (1) to arrange the source documents in the Documents section for use in the next step, that of constructing the Review Matrix, and (2) to provide a quick index for efficiently finding a particular source document at a later time. When you have reached the point of diminishing returns by apparently exhausting all of the references that can be added, and you have organized the Documents section in chronological order, you are ready to advance to the next step, that of constructing the Review Matrix. Bear in mind, however, that you probably will find more references and add more source materials to the Documents section while constructing the Review Matrix and even later while writing a synthesis of the literature.

HOW TO REMEMBER WHERE
YOU PUT THE DOCUMENTS

Losing track of where you stored your reprints is an occupational hazard. Researchers, policy analysts, science writers, and other professionals in the health sciences who systematically and critically review the literature on multiple subjects face this problem. Regardless of the scope of the tasks or the setting, everyone experiences the same problem—how to find their materials, even when the information is stored in a Lit Review Book. What is needed is some kind of tracking or indexing system.

In this section, a simple tracking system will be described that consists only of key words, references, and locations. A more sophisticated system, the Matrix Indexing System, is described in Chapter 8. The simple system, described here, will suffice to get you started.

Consider the following scenario: Your 3 Lit Review Books contain photocopies of 30 or 40 research studies in each of the Documents sections that you have assembled over considerable time and expense; you cannot remember the details of all of the reprints or even the key words; and you often need to find a specific paper in a hurry because of a report or grant deadline, a paper you are preparing, or a request from someone for information. Furthermore, the hours spent trying to find a copy of a document takes time away from the task you actually need to accomplish, such as completing the study or writing the report.

The key to quickly and efficiently accessing your own store of information is to create a tracking system. Suppose that you have added new source documents to the Documents section over the past several years, how do you remember what is there? What you need is a system that lists the contents of each Documents section. As part of that index, you could indicate which documents were used in the initial review. You could also index notes and other materials in the Paper Trail, but for the sake of simplicity, only the tracking of the Documents section will be described here.

One of the simplest ways to index the source documents is to keep a chronological list of references of the documents at the front of the Documents section. In other words, list each article or source document by its year of publication. Store this list on your computer or on a central server that can be accessed by a group of people. Each time a reprint is added in the Documents section, update the list.

A more sophisticated, high-tech strategy for indexing the contents of an expanding Documents section is the Matrix Indexing System, which is described in the next chapter. The low-tech approach is the tracking system described above that consists of a chronological list of reprints kept in a notebook or on a computer. Whichever system you use, the benefits accrue only if you keep the list up to date.

Caroline's Quest:
Assembling a Documents Section

Caroline's next task was to choose which of the 15 research articles she would abstract in the Review Matrix. First she sorted the papers by year of publication and began with the oldest paper, published in 1992. She read the abstract, and skimmed the entire paper, making notes in the margins of the papers she had photocopied about questions she would come back to later when she abstracted the final set of papers. At this point, Caroline was not doing any abstracting. In fact, she had not even decided which topics she would use as the basis for abstracting the studies. As she read, however, she made notes of potential topics for the Review Matrix. Of the 15 papers she scanned, Caroline chose 9 of the studies to include in the Documents section of her Lit Review Book on characteristics of adolescent girls who smoke.

"Well, that step was easy," Caroline commented to Professor Dickerson at their weekly meeting. She showed him her Lit Review Book with her notes in the Paper Trail section and the copies of the 9 articles in the Documents section.

"Yes, filing reprints is easy," Professor Dickerson agreed. "But your job isn't done yet. You need to constantly be alert for more studies as you read each of these articles. If you find that there are some authors who are referenced frequently, then look them up in *Science Citation Index* to see if you can find additional studies that also referenced them." He grinned. "Use the snowball technique to find more studies," he advised.

"What if I haven't found all the right studies?" Caroline looked concerned. "I could be missing something that is a classic in the field and not know it. Reviewing the literature seems like such a hit-or-miss kind of thing, even with the Matrix Method."

Professor Dickerson nodded, "I agree. You must constantly be looking for more studies. Abstracting the ones you have will probably help. You want to reach the point where you have the sense that you know who the researchers are and what research questions they have studied. In other words, you need to begin to own the literature."

"Okay, I understand how to use the documents. But what if all the documents I want to use have been gathered together already, say, in a special section in the library. Do I have to make a copy of each one and put them in a Documents section in order to do a review of the literature?" Caroline was thinking about the expense of all that photocopying.

"No," Professor Dickerson responded. "If the documents are available elsewhere and convenient to use, then, you don't have to copy them. The Documents section is meant to be a convenience for you and an organized way of maintaining a reprints file." He thought a minute, then continued, "Frankly, Caroline, I don't know of many situations in which all of the documents for a literature review have already been assembled in one place. You will also need to think about what to do with the articles themselves. One of the advantages of having a copy of an article when you abstract it for the Review Matrix is that you can mark it up as you read it. You can highlight certain key parts, or write questions to yourself in the margin of the paper, or turn your copy over and make notes on the back. If you are working from an original or a copy belonging to someone else or the library, then you can't mark it up."

He paused to let Caroline think about the pros and cons of making photocopies of the documents for her review, then he continued, "Now your task next week will be to read all of the articles and make some decisions about which column topics to use in your Review Matrix."

Review Matrix: How To Abstract the Research Literature

This chapter describes how to set up a Review Matrix, choose topics for the Matrix, and abstract each of the source documents based on these topics. The seven sections of this chapter are as follows:

- ☑ What Is a Review Matrix?
- ☑ How To Construct a Review Matrix
- ☑ How To Arrange Documents for Use in a Review Matrix
- ☑ How To Choose Column Topics for a Review Matrix
- ☑ How To Abstract Documents in a Review Matrix
- ☑ Fringe Benefits of the Abstracting Process
- ☑ Caroline's Quest: Constructing a Review Matrix

WHAT IS A REVIEW MATRIX?

A matrix is a box, with rows and columns, like a spreadsheet. In a Review Matrix the rows are for documents such as journal articles and the columns are for the topics you will use to abstract each of those documents. An abstract describes only the most pertinent points about the topic. Table 5-1 shows a generic example in which the first 2 rows are journal articles and the columns are the first 4 topics of the Review Matrix.

For example, if you were interested in abstracting an article by the famous Professor Brown on his (fictitious) paper, "The Cure for the Common Cold," the paper would be listed in the first row and the topics you are going to abstract about that paper would be listed across the top of the Review Matrix. Professor Brown's archrival, Professor White, published a similar paper in 1989, which you also abstracted. Table 5-2 illustrates how those 2 papers would look in the first part of a Review Matrix.

Table 5-1 Generic Review Matrix

Topic 1 Example: Author, title, journal	Topic 2 Example: Year	Topic 3 Example: Purpose	Topic 4 Example: Type of Study Design
Journal article 1	1995	Drug treatment for epilepsy	Experimental study
Journal article 2	1997	Drug treatment for depression	Case-control study

---

Thus, a Review Matrix is a rectangular arrangement, or a matrix, in which the rows always have the journal articles or papers listed down the side and the topics or issues you are going to abstract for each article are always listed across the top.

Advantages of a Review Matrix

The reason for using the Matrix Method is to create order out of chaos. In a review of the literature, the chaos you must

Table 5-2 Review Matrix for Literature on Cure for the Common Cold

Author, Title, Journal	Year	Purpose	Methodological Design
Brown, C.J. Cure for the common cold. Journal of Scientific Wonder.	1987	Compare drug X with a placebo for cold cure	Randomized clinical trial
White, R.M. A better cure for the common cold. Journal of Better Science.	1989	Compare drug Y with drug X for superior cold cure	Randomized clinical trial

deal with is too much information spread across too many journal articles or other source documents with too many details to remember. The order you are going to impose is that of organizing all this information so you can then think about it and use it efficiently. The Review Matrix provides a standard structure for creating order. Constructing a Review Matrix is like building a house. You will still need to furnish the house, in this case by reading and abstracting each article and putting that information in each cell, but the Review Matrix provides a "place for everything" which allows you to efficiently and reliably concentrate on the information itself.

HOW TO CONSTRUCT A REVIEW MATRIX

Constructing a Review Matrix as a basis for writing a synthesis in a literature review is a simple 3-step process:

1. **Organizing the documents.** Organize the Documents section chronologically by arranging the source documents from the oldest to the most recent by year of publication.
2. **Choosing topics.** Set up the Review Matrix, either on paper or electronically in a word processor or spreadsheet, and decide which topics to use for this review of the literature.

3. **Abstracting the documents.** Read and abstract each source document one at a time in chronological order, from oldest to most recent, and record your notes under each topic in the Review Matrix.

HOW TO ARRANGE DOCUMENTS FOR USE IN A REVIEW MATRIX

Source documents should be organized chronologically, from the oldest to the most recent by year of publication. Most of the source documents you will abstract in the Review Matrix probably will be research papers and other journal articles or book chapters. Most of the documents will be stored in the Documents section of your Lit Review Book, as discussed in Chapter 4.

HOW TO CHOOSE COLUMN TOPICS FOR A REVIEW MATRIX

What Is a Column Topic?

In a review of the literature, the 3 most important decisions you will make are (1) specifying the purpose of the literature review, (2) selecting the source documents, and (3) choosing the column topics. Column topics in a Review Matrix are the issues or concepts used to abstract each journal article or other source document in a review of the literature.

For example, if one of the column topics is "sampling design," then your task in completing a Review Matrix is to identify the type of design used to select subjects for every study abstracted. If the authors did not describe the sampling design, then record its absence in that study by noting that it is not available (N.A.) or give your best guess, for example, "NA— probably volunteer subjects."

Categories of Column Topics

Rarely will a review of the literature be so comprehensive as to include all of the column topics possible. When reviewing the scientific literature, consider 2 broad categories in thinking about the column topics you choose: (1) methodological characteristics of the study, and (2) content-specific characteristics such as the theoretical or conceptual model, the types of results, or the implications for policy.

Most studies published in scientific journals in the health and behavior literature follow a standard format, as described in the section on Anatomy of a Scientific Paper in Chapter 2, and include a common set of methodological characteristics describing how the study was designed and analyzed. In choosing column topics, consider including some of these methodological characteristics. A list of methodological topics and a description of each are described in Guidelines for a Methodological Review of the Literature in Chapter 2.

Because these methodological topics will not be sufficient to describe a body of research, be sure to include topics that cover the content of the research. Choose topics based on their relevance to the purpose of your literature review.

First Three Column Topics

Make it a practice to always let the first 3 columns in any Review Matrix be the same. Use these 3 columns to record fundamental information about each source document you abstract:

- Column 1: Author(s), title, name of journal
- Column 2: Year of publication
- Column 3: Purpose of the paper or source document

In the first column, record all of the names of multiple authors of a paper or book, not just the first 3 followed by et al. By including all authors, you will be in a better position to track all of the researchers involved in this kind of research. Look for the same researchers as authors of other papers later in time, whether or not they published together.

Setting aside a column for the year is important because that is the basis on which you will sort and index all source documents as well as the reprints in the Documents section. Year of publication is the key to quickly and efficiently finding photo-copies of articles.

The third column is set aside to describe the purpose of the document—why was the study done or what was the purpose of the document? State the purpose in your own words. For a research study, try to describe the purpose as a research question. If you (or the authors of the paper) cannot describe the intended purpose in the form of a question, how can you (or they) know if the question was answered? Describing the purpose may be difficult at times. Some authors do not provide a clear statement of purpose in the Introduction section of a paper, and you may have to read the entire paper in order to determine what they intended to do.

The choice of the rest of the topics is up to you. This is a judgment call that will be based on the purpose of your literature review and your knowledge about the topic. While there are no rules for generating a list of topics or choosing among them, what follows are some suggestions for a process that may be useful.

Process for Choosing the Remaining Topics

What if you don't know what topics to choose, other than the first 3? Even if you are doing a literature review to find out something about the latest research in an unfamiliar field, you do know something about the topic. By the time you are ready to choose the column topics for a Review Matrix, you will have consulted reference books about the topic, read numerous abstracts on an electronic bibliographic database or in journals, and skimmed the papers of the source documents selected for the Documents section. The 4-step process to use in deciding which column topics to include is summarized below.

Step 1—Read the Documents. Read all of the articles or source documents in the Documents Section in chronological order so that you can grasp the scope of the research. This will also begin to give you a sense of how the research issues and methodologies have changed over time. For this second brief reading of the articles, the purpose is to gain enough of a perspective to choose column topics.

Step 2—List Important Issues. While reading the source documents, make a list of the most important issues, both methodological as well as content-specific. For example, if some of the earlier studies used observational designs, but later ones used experimental designs, then type of methodological design might be an important topic. Alternatively, if the area you are reviewing is limited to Medicare recipients, then you might make a note of that but not devote a column to a topic that will be true for all studies.

Step 3—Select Column Topics. Once you have finished reading all of the source documents, select the topics that seem to be the most important from 2 standpoints: issues in the field and the purpose of your literature review. For example, suppose that you are reviewing the literature on worldwide epidemiology of HIV and are especially interested in the rates in South American countries compared to other parts of the world. With regard to content, you might set aside a column for how HIV status was assessed in each study. For purposes of your review, you might include another column for the country in which the subjects resided.

Step 4—Add Column Topics. After you have begun to abstract the first few source documents, you may need to add some important topics. Plan for this addition in advance by leaving some blank columns in the Review Matrix. (This is easier if done on a computer spreadsheet.) Additional topics can be added at any time. Be sure to go back and include the papers you have already abstracted when you add those topics. Sometimes it is not possible to know the full range of topics until you have abstracted all of the documents. (If that happens, then the philosophy of the Review Matrix is working: the abstracting process enabled you to identify an important topic that you hadn't seen when you began.) Add the missing topics and abstract all the papers again on that basis.

A Matter of Thoroughness

At this point, you may be thinking that this amount of detail and effort require too much commitment on your part, especially when your counterparts have already accomplished their review of the literature in a tenth of the time by simply going to the library with a stack of index cards, reading the journal articles once without going to the trouble (or expense) of making photocopies, and writing their summary of the literature. Whether or not to proceed is fundamentally a decision that only you can make. Think about why you are doing a review of the literature and what the consequences will be of not doing it thoroughly. If you are trying to understand what is known about a specific subject or if you want to identify what is missing in a body of research, then you must own the literature. Can you take the chance that you have overlooked an important paper? Are you willing to design your own research study without knowing whether or not some other researcher already has addressed that very question? How thorough is thorough enough?

There is no thoroughness index that will tell you when you have done enough. Your only guide to determining thoroughness is your own sense of knowing the literature well enough—to own it. The Matrix Method is one way of approaching that type of ownership, but it is not a guarantee of thoroughness. Should you decide to continue, the next step is to concentrate on a single article or paper at a time, read it thoroughly and abstract it based on the column topics. Then read and abstract the next source document until all have been examined.

HOW TO ABSTRACT DOCUMENTS
IN A REVIEW MATRIX

Taking Notes

What do you do when you abstract an article? At the simplest level, you write down a note about the topic in the area, or cell, where the row and column meet in the Review Matrix. By now, you have read each article at least twice, first to decide whether or not to make a photocopy to include in the Documents section, and second to make a decision about which column topics to use. Next comes the third and most intensive reading in which you will critically analyze the source materials, abstract each on the basis of the column topics, and in the process, construct the cells of the Review Matrix.

Essential Tools. Never read an empirical paper without a calculator. Check the numbers and the percentages. Do the number of subjects in the tables of results add up to the numbers the researchers said they enrolled at the beginning of the study? All of this will help you understand what the authors did in conducting their study. Two other important tools to have at hand when critically reading a research paper are a highlighter for marking important sections of the paper and a pencil for writing notes and questions on the paper itself.

Recreate the Study in Your Mind

Be forewarned that simply recording information in the Review Matrix without reconstructing the study in your own mind does not really constitute a critical review of the literature. In order to thoroughly read a scientific paper, you must essentially re-create the study by retracing the authors' steps. Begin by asking yourself questions such as, what was their purpose, how did they go about doing the study, what were their results, and what was their logic in their interpretation of the results they found? In the process of understanding what the authors did, determine whether or not you agree scientifically with their purpose, methods, results, and interpretations. That is the critical part of critically reviewing the literature.

In one sense, each scientific paper is a story, a true story, and you have to accurately tell that story in your own words in order to fully understand the paper. Make notes in the margins of the paper as you read it, circle words you don't understand or terms the authors didn't define and look them up, highlight important parts of the paper such as the purpose or key results, and draw diagrams of the time relationships. For example, when was the pretest administered, how much later was the intervention, how long did the intervention last, and how long after that was the post-test?

Read in Chronological Order

The chronological order in which you read the papers is also important. Begin with the oldest paper, based on its publication date, and end with the most recent. The reason for reading in chronological order is that the research of later papers should build on the results of a previous body of work. Perhaps the findings of 1 paper suggested a new theory for a future study, a new analytic method became available, or an old study was reanalyzed.

Of course the progress you may see over time depends on the range of papers selected for your review, and there may be gaps in the progression of the science because of papers you overlooked or decided not to analyze. If this appears to be the case, you can always go back and include the missing articles.

Write Notes in the Matrix

In constructing a Review Matrix, your task is to take each article or source material and record notes based on the column topics. The notes in the cells of the Review Matrix have to be concise and very short. Their purpose is to allow you to track the details of a study, not to summarize the entire article.

Occasionally, you will have included an article that is a review of other studies or a theoretical paper. In this case, you might want to ignore the column topics and make a note in the Review Matrix for that row about the importance of that paper or whether it is a good summary.

Other papers may include important points or quotes that you will want to remember without having to search back through all of the materials in the Documents section. Write these more detailed notes on the back (the blank side) of the

Review Matrix sheet (or elsewhere on a computer file) and make a note in the matrix that further information has been recorded.

An example of the process of reading a research paper in preparation for abstracting it in the Review Matrix is shown in Exhibit 5-1.

Additional Information

In the meantime, as you read each source document, add to your list of references and photocopy additional articles that will be added to the Documents section, as needed. Not everything will fit neatly under one of the column topics. If you are using a large sheet of paper, leave the backside blank, and use it for additional notes. If you are using a spreadsheet or word processor, set aside a special section or file to include these notes. Remember to plan for expansion. If your Review Matrix is on paper rather than a computer, then begin a new year at the top of each page of the matrix so that you can insert additional articles in the future.

FRINGE BENEFITS OF THE ABSTRACTING PROCESS

Overview

The reason for constructing a Review Matrix is to provide a basis for systematically analyzing the literature and writing a review of the literature in the form of a synthesis. Constructing a Review Matrix is both tedious and time-consuming, but there are some additional advantages in the abstracting process itself, provided you have done a thorough job of collecting the most relevant research papers on a subject. In the first place, you learn something about the sociology of the subject you are reviewing. Second, by taking apart and abstracting each study using the same set of topics, you are better able to state questions of your own. Finally, you begin to have a better sense of what is missing and areas in which new research is needed.

Exhibit 5-1 How To Abstract a Research Paper

INTRODUCTION SECTION

Begin with the Introduction section of the paper. Rephrase the authors' purpose in your own words. Put it in the form of a research question. If the authors haven't included a purpose—some don't—then state what you think their question is, and make a note that they did not state the purpose.

METHODS SECTION

Read and reread each part of the Methods section of the paper until you have a clear idea of what the authors did. Sometimes authors (or editors) leave out important information. If so, describe what you think they did—but make a note that this was your opinion. In order to really understand the study, you need to re-create what the authors did in carrying it out. In other words, describe for yourself the procedures they used.

Now look at the numbers in the subsection about subjects and how they were selected for the study. Begin with the number of subjects—is it possible to trace how many were in the sample at the beginning of the study and how many subjects were lost as the study progressed? Subjects get lost for a variety of reasons: they might have died or moved away or simply may not have responded. This is where your calculator comes in. Figure out what the real response rate was; don't depend on the authors' calculations.

The reason this response rate is so important is that researchers run the risk of subject bias if the characteristics of the sample of subjects who end the study differ from those who began the study. For example, the authors may report that the response rate to a questionnaire was 87% (that is, 87% of the people who were asked to fill out the questionnaire actually did) or that the completion rate for an intervention was 45%. Anything less than 100% raises the possibility of a sample bias, but a rate alone does not indicate sample bias. The authors must compare the people who did and did not respond, and then describe in the paper what the differences were statistically. Many authors do not include that information. If they haven't in-

continues

Exhibit 5-1 continued

cluded it, then make a note of this potential weakness of the study.

Now take this same critical approach to reading about how the data were collected. Was a questionnaire or survey used? If so, what questions or items were included? Was research completed on the instrument itself before it was used in this study? For example, what do the authors report about the validity and reliability of the instrument? If data from a national study were used, then have the authors provided references so you can go back and get the information about how the data were collected? Don't automatically assume that a study was done correctly just because a national sample of subjects was drawn or this was part of a very large project. Read critically.

Continue to read each part of the Methods section of the paper in this way. If you don't know what to look for, review the section on Guidelines for a Methodological Review in Chapter 2.

RESULTS SECTION

Reread the purpose of the paper, then examine the results section to see if the authors answered the research questions or hypotheses they initially stated. Were additional questions posed and answered in the process of addressing the main questions? Were there additional research questions that were not answered?

DISCUSSION SECTION

As you read the paper, think about the strengths and weaknesses of the study, and then note whether or not the authors described the same problems or advantages. Note especially what additional research questions were not addressed. Ask yourself what the implications of the results were or the significance of these findings.

continues

Exhibit 5-1 continued

REFERENCES

You might find it useful to make notes about the references at the end of each paper. Specifically, go through the references of each paper and add to your own list (in the Paper Trail section) any that call for follow-up.

ACKNOWLEDGMENTS

This column topic might be included in the review if issues such as funding source are relevant. For example, you might consider whether or not the funding source of a research project posed a potential conflict of interest, such as a study about the rates of teenage smoking that has been funded by the tobacco industry.

REVIEWER-SPECIFIC TOPICS

A Review Matrix should be tailored to the purpose of your review of the literature. Rarely will a review be so comprehensive as to include all of the column topics described above. In fact, you may choose to include only a few of the topics described above and instead opt for some very specific topics of your own. For example, if your review of the literature is limited to experimental studies, then it might be redundant to have a column topic on experimental designs. Alternatively, if you believe that knowing which kinds of experimental designs would be important to understanding this literature, then you will need such a column topic. These reviewer-specific column topics may dominate the review of the literature, to the exclusion of many of the other topics listed above.

SOME GENERAL ADVICE

Rarely will you ever read straight through a paper in a linear fashion, from Introduction to the Discussion section. You may start out this way, but as you get into the paper, you will find it

continues

Exhibit 5-1-continued

necessary to go back and recheck some of the details. For example, in the midst of the Methods section you may jump ahead to the Results section ("Did they really keep all of the subjects in the study who were enrolled at the beginning?") or in the middle of reading about the results, you may return to the Introduction section ("What did the authors say the purpose was?"). As you read these papers, keep a running dialogue with yourself about what the researchers intended to do, what they really did, what they reported they found, and what they actually found.

This double-checking is important. Don't assume anything, and don't give any author of a research paper the benefit of the doubt. In reviewing the literature, the best attitude is to be methodologically suspicious and ever-doubtful.

Sociology of the Research Topic

As you carefully read and abstract each source document in chronological order, especially if they are research papers in a specific area, then you will begin to know

- who the researchers are and who they collaborate with,
- where the research is being done,
- whether or not they tend to use the same datasets,
- what the funding sources are, and
- which studies are cited repeatedly.

In other words, without consciously trying to, you begin to become aware of the sociology of this research topic as you abstract the studies.

Who the Researchers Are. Knowing the names of the researchers is useful if you want to find related studies by running an author search on MEDLINE or one of the other electronic bibliographic databases. *Science Citation Index* is a useful source for finding other studies by authors not included in the group now familiar to you. Knowing who collaborates with whom is important when learning about a new research field. For example, what appears to be a widespread research effort being done by a multitude of different researchers may, upon closer inspection, be the product of the same group or sub-group of collaborators who happen to be located in diverse university and nonacademic settings. There is nothing wrong with such an effort, in fact it has become even more feasible with the advent of the Internet. Such information would be useful if you wanted to contact someone in that group and discovered that one of them was in your institution or a place nearby.

Where the Research is Done. In the process of abstracting, you will begin to notice where the authors are located geographically. Some research efforts take place in a single institution, others, as suggested above, may be spread throughout the country. For example, most of the work in the area of evidence-based medicine was done at McMaster University, although there were some collaborators in other Canadian and American universities. If you were interested in pursuing that topic in greater depth, going to McMaster or contacting someone there might be the first place to start. Checking out the group's web site for a list of current or prospective publications would also be useful.

Datasets They Have in Common. Often, researchers in a related area use the same dataset, such as one of the National Health Interview Surveys (NHIS)[1-3] or the National Health and Nutrition Examination Survey (NHANES). If you are familiar with how the data were gathered and what the strengths and limitations of these datasets are, then you are in a better position to evaluate the studies that used them. To locate studies based on these large-scale, nationally representative databases, use the database name, such as NHANES, as a key word search on MEDLINE. More information about the databases can be obtained at the web site of the Department of Health and Human Services, http://www.os.dhhs.gov/.

Funding Sources. If 2 or more studies have been funded by the same source, you might find research projects in the same area by looking up that funding source. For example, if a study has been funded by a research grant from the National Institute on Aging, then do a CRISP search on the NIH database on the Internet to see if additional studies have been funded. (See Chapter 3 for information about how to conduct a CRISP search.) Some of the more recently funded studies still may be in progress and the results will not have been published yet. It is also possible that some of currently funded projects are being done by researchers other than those whose papers you have read, and they may be exploring different aspects of what is currently being published. In this case, consider contacting the principal investigators of these ongoing studies to find out something about their work. Whether or not you choose to take this extra step depends on why you are doing this review of the literature. Many private foundations also list research projects they have funded in the past or are currently funding. Look them up on the Internet.

Same Basic References. When checking the references section at the end of most research papers published in health sciences journals, you may find that the same set of research papers are being cited repeatedly by the authors of the documents you are abstracting. If you haven't included these papers in your own review, consider adding them to the ones you are abstracting.

Seeing What Is Missing

As you abstract each of the studies in your literature review, you are better able to develop your own questions about the research issues. Finding the answers to these questions will enable you to see the bigger picture. There is a real advantage for the person writing a grant proposal to see where the holes are in the current research on a topic. The abstracting process makes it possible for you to begin to see not only the issues that apparently have not been addressed but many of the methodological flaws as well. Discovering what is missing is part of owning the literature, and constructing the Review Matrix makes this possible.

Caroline's Quest:
Constructing a Review Matrix

Once Caroline had arranged the reprints chronologically in the Documents section of her Lit Review Book, she was ready to choose the column topics for the Review Matrix. She reread each of the research papers quickly and jotted down further notes about which issues or topics appeared to be the most important. She also reviewed the list of methodological topics (as described in Chapter 2) that Professor Dickerson had given her. She knew that she would not need all of the methodological topics, but some of them probably would be useful.

Caroline began by listing the first 3 topics that were standard in every Review Matrix constructed using the Matrix Method: (1) authors, title, and journal; (2) year of publication; and (3) purpose. Next, she decided to concentrate on some of the methodological characteristics, in her column topics, and for that reason she chose the outcome variable, which she recorded as the "dependent variable" in the Review Matrix. She knew that the studies varied in their definition of smoking. Depending on the purpose of each study, some authors concentrated only on cigarette smoking; others included chewing tobacco.

The next column topic she wrote down was "independent variable." This was the topic that would help her sort out which characteristics the authors had used to look at variations in smoking behavior. Caroline continued to add topics, such as the number of subjects in the study and whether or not the study was limited to females only or included both sexes.

Altogether, Caroline chose 17 topics, which she listed across the top of her still blank Review Matrix. Eleven of those topics are shown in Exhibit 5-2, which lists only the methodological topics plus a comment topic, which she reserved for making notes about the strengths and weaknesses of each study.

Caroline left several columns blank so that she could add a few additional topics as she abstracted the studies. She was ready to begin to abstract the studies she had chosen.

Caroline began the abstracting process by setting aside the Review Matrix, taking out her calculator and a yellow highlighter, and turning to the first paper in the

Exhibit 5-2 Caroline's Review Matrix for Research Literature on Smoking by Adolescent Girls

continues

Author Title, Journal	Year Pub	PURPOSE	VARIABLES		SUBJECTS			DATA		COMMENTS
			Dependent	Independent	# of Ss	Subject characteristics	Sample Design	Source or Instrument	Yr data collect	
Wang, Fitzhugh, Westerfield, Eddy. Family & peer influences on smoking behavior among Americ. adolescents: an age trend. *Soc of Adoles Med.*	1995	What is influence of family and peers on adolescent smoking?	cigarette smoking only	peer by sex family—sibling, father, mother	6,900	male & female, 14-18 yrs	nat'l—random (82% responserate)	Nat'l Hlth Interv Surv	1988-89	• no response/non resp analysis for Ss • no info on data collect instrument • no race irformation
Altman, Levine, Coeytaux, Slade, Jaffe. Tobacco promotion use among adol. aged 12–17 years in a natl repres. sample. *AJPH.*	1996	What is relation between youth susceptibility to tobacco use and participation in promotional campaign?	suscep to tob: • non-tob use • suscep to tobac • current tob. use cigarette & chew tobacco	age, gender, tob. user in household, awareness of tob promot, know friend owns promot item, particip in tob promot, mail from tob, free sample	1,047	male & female, 12–17 yrs	nat'l—random (62% response rate)	author conduct sample—random digit dialing across U.S.	1993	• no resp/non-resp analysis • no infor on data collection instrum • no race info

Exhibit 5-2 continued

Author Title, Journal	Year Pub	PURPOSE	VARIABLES		SUBJECTS			DATA			COMMENTS
			Dependent	Independent	# of Ss	Subject characteristics	Sample Design	Source or Instrument	Yr data collect		
French & Perry. Smoking among adolescent girls; prevalence & etiology. *JAMWA*.	1996	To review lit on prevalence & etiology of smok by adolescent girls.	cigarette smoking	female, race	varies by study	female, 17–18 yrs	across multiple studies	varies	varies		Not an empirical study. Summary of literature only. • info on race included. Note prevalence rates.

Documents section. *This was the third time she had read this paper, but this was the most concentrated reading. Caroline highlighted the sentence in the Purpose section of the paper and she wrote down the dependent and independent variables in the margins of the paper. She used her calculator to track the percentage of subjects who dropped out of the study or who did not respond to the survey. Caroline continued to read the paper thoroughly until she had a clear understanding of what the purpose of the study was, how the authors had conducted the study, and what they had found.*

Then Caroline turned to the Review Matrix and began to make notes for that study under each of the column topics. After examining the list of references at the end of the paper, she added a few references to her list to look up in MEDLINE when she finished abstracting.

Caroline abstracted each paper immediately after reading it. Examples of 3 of the papers she abstracted, the Wang et al. study,[4] the Altman et al. paper,[5] and the French and Perry article[6] are shown in Exhibit 5-2. Although the paper by French and Perry was not an actual study, it was important because it was a thorough review of the literature on the prevalence and etiology of smoking by adolescent girls and included 35 references that might provide further resources. Caroline included this paper and made a note in the comments column that the authors had reported rates of smoking for teenage girls.

When Caroline finished abstracting all of the articles in the Documents section of her Lit Review Book, she took the list of additional references she had compiled during the abstracting process and looked each up on MEDLINE. She then repeated the process she had followed earlier of considering whether or not to include any of these papers in her review. A paper published in 1993 was added. Caroline included this study in the Review Matrix at the end of the 1993 list and abstracted it as she had done the others.

Upon completion, Caroline had a Review Matrix filled in with notes for each article. The Matrix was a little messy because there were additional notes on the back and a few more column topics had been added. She was now ready to write the synthesis.

REFERENCES

1. National Center for Health Statistics. *Health Interview Survey Procedures, 1957–1974.* Hyattsville, MD: US Department of Health, Education, and Welfare, Public Health Service, Health Resources Administration; 1975.
2. Kovar MG, Poe GS. *The National Health Interview Survey Design, 1975–83.* Hyattsville, MD: US Department of Health and Human Services, Public Health Service, National Center for Health Statistics; 1985.
3. Masey JT, Moore TF, Parsons VL, Tadros W. *Design and Estimation for the National Health Interview Survey, 1985–94.* Hyattsville, MD: US Department of Health and Human Services, Public Health Service, Center for Disease Control, National Center for Health Statistics; 1989.
4. Wang MQ, Fitzhugh EC, Westerfield RC, Eddy JM. Family and peer influences on smoking behavior among American adolescents: An age trend. *Journal of Adolescent Health.* 1995;16:200–203.
5. Altman DG, Levine DW, Coeytaux R, Slade J, Jaffe R. Tobacco promotion and susceptibility to tobacco use among adolescents aged 12 through 17 years in a nationally representative sample. *AJPH.* 1996;86:1590–1593.
6. French SA, Perry CL. Smoking among adolescent girls: Prevalence and etiology. *Journal of the American Medical Womens Association.* 1996; 51:25–28.

Synthesis: How To Use a Review Matrix To Write a Synthesis

The goal of a review of the literature is to summarize your critical analysis about the research literature on a specific topic in the form of a narrative. This chapter describes how to use a Review Matrix to write such a synthesis and includes the following sections:

- ☑ What Is a Synthesis?
- ☑ How To Use a Review Matrix To Write a Synthesis
- ☑ Caroline's Quest: Writing a Synthesis

135

WHAT IS A SYNTHESIS?

A synthesis is a critical analysis and review of the scientific literature on a specific topic. Unlike a summary of different articles, a synthesis is based on the same set of papers and examines the themes of the research as they have developed across the studies and over the years, including similarities and discrepancies in content, methodology, and findings. A synthesis also examines the literature for what is missing—where the holes are in both the content and the research methodology. The goal of a synthesis is to critically analyze the content of the research, research methodologies, and results, and then to pull the disparate parts together into a logical coherent whole.

Advantages of a Synthesis

Most people find that they do not formulate interpretations or opinions about the research studies until they have written a systematic review of the literature. A well-written literature review requires that you complete 2 major tasks: critically analyze the literature and write a synthesis. The operational word here is *write.* To stop before putting the synthesis into written form will have accomplished only half the task of your literature review.

What This Chapter Does Not Cover

This chapter is not about how to write. There are excellent books available on that subject, beginning with the classic, *If You Want to Write,* by Brenda Ueland.[1] Other excellent guides are *How to Write: Advice and Reflections* by Pulitzer Prize winning writer, Richard Rhodes,[2] and *Writing Down the Bones* by award winning writing instructor, Natalie Goldberg.[3] You will also need a good grammar book. The classic is *Elements of Style* by Strunk and White;[4] its witty, contemporary counterpart is *Woe is I* by Patricia O'Conner.[5] These writing and grammar books are excellent resources, whether you intend to write a synthesis of the literature or any other kind of document.

HOW TO USE A REVIEW MATRIX TO WRITE A SYNTHESIS

The Tools You Will Need

Once all of the source documents in the Documents section have been abstracted and the Review Matrix has been completed, you are ready to begin the synthesis. The Review Matrix is the primary tool for organizing and writing the synthesis. You will use not only the content in the matrix, but also the tracking information to quickly locate the original articles in the Documents section. Thus, you will need both the Review Matrix and the Documents section close at hand in writing the synthesis.

Using the Review Matrix

The Review Matrix has a different use in writing a synthesis than it did for abstracting source documents. Constructing the Review Matrix required you to develop the rows of the matrix by analyzing one study at a time based on the column topics. In writing a synthesis of the literature, you will focus on the columns of the Review Matrix as you compare the studies.

Of course you have to know each of the studies, but when you begin to synthesize them, you are looking at them from a different angle. For example, you could think about how the studies varied over time in their use of a particular theory. Alternatively, you might want to identify only those studies that included both male and female subjects. By scanning down a particular column of the Review Matrix, you can readily identify those studies. (This would be easier on a computer with a sorting capability for each of the columns.) You might also look for the lack of something across the studies. For example, in papers on the epidemiology of epilepsy, did any of the subject populations include people over 65 years of age? If you abstracted information in the Review Matrix about subjects' age ranges, then you will be able to look for that possibility. In general, as you critically evaluate the different studies, think about the underlying factor you want to use to show variations or lack thereof over time.

Reason for the Review

The first step in writing a synthesis is to be clear about why you are doing a literature review. The most common reasons for reviewing the literature include summarizing previous scholarly work for a paper or report for a class, background material for a presentation or publication; a thesis or dissertation required in a graduate program; a research proposal, including a request for grant or contract funds; and a scientific article, possibly describing your own research or that of others.

The focus of the literature review will vary, depending on the reason for doing the review. The reason should provide you with guidance in focusing the literature review. In a thesis or dissertation, the Previous Research section contains most of the review of the literature, while the Background and Significance section of a standard grant or contract proposal includes most of the literature review. In the thesis or dissertation and the research proposal, the review of the literature may focus not only on the major topic, such as previous research on the effects of poor nutrition among lower income children, but also on a methodological review, that is, the types of research methods used by previous researchers in the field to investigate that topic. In a scientific paper, the review of the literature will be most evident in the Introduction and Discussion sections.

Define the Purpose of the Review

The next step in writing a synthesis is to clearly define the purpose of the review of the literature. You should have done this already when you began assembling the Paper Trail; however, that purpose may have changed as you read and reread the source documents. Perhaps the purpose is more refined in scope or has been expanded to encompass more issues. Either way, the first working sentence of your synthesis should be, "The purpose of this review of the literature is. . . ."

Describe the Search and Review Process

Describe briefly the strategy used to select and review the documents included in your literature review. This description provides basic information about your search and selection process, such as the period of time covered by the review; the sources used, including electronic bibliographic database and journals; types of articles; and the conditions for inclusions and exclusions. The following example conveys such information:

> The review of the literature covered a 10-year period, from 1990 to 1999. The search included use of 3 electronic bibliographic databases, MEDLINE, Health-STAR, and International Pharmaceutical Abstracts, with special attention to the leading clinical journals in this area (*Journal of X, Journal of Y,* and *Journal of Z*). Only empirical studies were reviewed; letters to the editor, policy statements, and program descriptions were excluded. A total of 103 papers were examined, of which 23 met the criteria.

Because you are using the Matrix Method, you might also tell the reader what topics were used to abstract the documents. Here is an example:

> Using the Matrix Method,[6] each of the 23 papers was evaluated in ascending chronological order using a structured abstracting form with 12 topics: journal identification, purpose, definition of independent and dependent variables, covariates, methodological design, sampling design, number of subjects, respondent/nonrespondent analysis, data sources, validity and reliability of data collection, results, and significance.

The description of the search and abstracting process will vary, depending on the purpose of your review. For example, if you are summarizing the literature for a research paper, then the description may need to be more concise. Alternatively, the process used to review the literature for a meta-analysis will need to be more extensive. Regardless of the purpose of your paper, a statement of the search and abstracting process will give the reader a sense of the thoroughness of your literature review.

List the Principal Topics

Now think about which topics you will use to organize the synthesis. A thorough synthesis of the literature includes a discussion of 1 or more of the following:

- **Issues**—the major reasons or problems that motivated this body of research, including the theoretical or conceptual models and the hypothesis or research question
- **Methods**—the research methods used to investigate the problems, including 1 or more of the column topics, are listed under the broad headings of methodology, data collection instruments and procedures, subjects, and data analysis
- **Results**—the major findings or results
- **Missing or inadequate topics**—the topics or issues that are missing, that is, those that have not been investigated at all or have been covered inadequately
- **Critical analysis**—your critical analysis of each of these sections.

It is important to separate your discussion of the literature, that is, the issues, methods, results, and missing topics, from your critical analysis. Make certain that you specify which is which in your review. Although all 5 issues are needed, your critical analysis of this body of research is probably the most important. *Critical,* in this context, is not the same as negative. A critical analysis is one in which you have weighed all the evidence and made an informed judgment about the adequacy, appropriateness, and thoroughness of the studies reviewed.

You can structure the written synthesis of the literature in several different ways. One approach might be to write up each of the first 4 sections—issues, methods, missing or inadequate, results—and at the end of each of those sections give a critical analysis.

Another approach would be to summarize the first 4 topics together and conclude with a section containing the critical analysis. Often, the decision about how to structure a review of the literature will be made after you have written the first draft, not at the beginning of the process. In fact, you may choose the structure only after revising the review several times.

Alternatively, the reason for doing the review may dictate the structure and format of your synthesis. For example, a synthesis written for a doctoral dissertation will be very different from one prepared for a research study manuscript being submitted to a peer-reviewed journal.

Read Down the Columns

With the purpose, topics, and structure of your written synthesis in mind, how do you use the Review Matrix to synthesize the information? Read each of the columns of the matrix, from top to bottom, and determine what happened within each topic heading across the studies and over time. For example, if you are summarizing the themes of the research studies, look down the Purpose column in the Review Matrix. Are there specific issues that appear, disappear, and then reappear over the years?

If it is necessary to gather more details, go back and reread some of the papers, which you already will have arranged in convenient, chronological order, in the Documents section of the Lit Review Book. Having abstracted all of the articles, you should have developed a sense of how thoroughly the various authors reviewed other studies by their inclusion of citations to published papers. Did these authors refer to other studies? Alternatively, did other authors seem to strike out on their own, without referring to the work of previous research that could have been used to better develop their own ideas? Taken as a body of research, does this collection of articles suggest that many different themes were addressed over the past decade, or does this set of articles focus on one central theme, with the studies building on one another?

Do the papers seem to concentrate on increasingly specific details about the same issue, with only a few that explore new areas of inquiry? Is this an appropriate, creative, or necessary diversion from the mainstream of research on the subject? If you are developing ideas for your own research, perhaps in the form of a dissertation or research proposal, what holes are there that you might focus on in this body of research?

The same kind of thinking could be applied to the methodologies used to examine the research questions. Are the studies merely descriptive, or do subsequent studies describe innovative approaches for solving the problem? For example, in the research literature on falls among elderly women, initial papers described high prevalence rates that often resulted in the women's confinement to a nursing home or in their death. Later papers reported a statistical association between falls and antianxiety drugs, with the conclusion that these medications were overused in the elderly population. In subsequent papers, only a subclass of antianxiety drugs was found to be the problem. Next was a series of studies that described the effects of different methods for intervening with practicing physicians to convince them to change their prescription of these drugs, especially for older people. Taken as a whole, this body of research moved from the initial description of the problem, through association with risk factors, to intervention. The corresponding methodological designs used in these studies followed a similar progression: from descriptive to quasi-experimental to experimental designs.

Upon completing the synthesis, you will need to store a written copy of your review of the literature in the Synthesis section of the Lit Review Book for later reference. Consider storing an electronic copy on the hard disk of your computer.

Caroline's Quest:
Writing a Synthesis

Caroline met with Professor Dickerson to go over her Review Matrix and discuss the next steps. "Keep in mind why you are writing this synthesis," Professor Dickerson cautioned her, "The way you write the review, its length, and issues you cover may vary depending on whether the synthesis is being written for a term paper, a thesis, or a grant proposal. In this case, you know it is the introductory section for your thesis, but in the future, your purpose will vary."

Caroline understood his point, but had a question about her immediate task, "I'd like to talk about how to organize the synthesis itself. You know, what do I discuss first, then next, and so forth?"

Professor Dickerson nodded and said, "I know what you mean. The first thing to remember is that you should not merely summarize each paper. Think about the issues you want to describe. Certainly you will be referring to and describing information from each study, but your focus should be on a critical analysis of the major aspects of research that these studies cover. You might begin your synthesis by describing the purpose of your review and limitations that you chose, such as a focus on adolescent girls between the ages of 13 and 18 years old. You could also include a few sentences on the search itself, the years you restricted it to, the databases you searched, and the number of articles you included in the review. All of this is preliminary to your actual synthesis, however, and should probably not take more that half a page. Concentrate the remainder of your synthesis on the critical analysis of the studies."

"For example," he continued, "think about the different kinds of research questions that the authors asked in their studies. Were there any major themes? If so, describe them briefly. Summarize the major findings, and then discuss how the studies differed in what they found. In general, think about using the following strategy: summarize the issue, describe variations across the studies, discuss strengths and weaknesses of the studies, and give your interpretation about what this means."

Caroline looked at the materials she had brought with her. "So how do I use the Review Matrix in writing the synthesis?" she asked. "Or is preparing the Review Matrix just a way of making me read each article in a disciplined fashion?"

"Good question," Professor Dickerson responded. "You're right, filling in the Review Matrix does make you read each study carefully and make notes on the same set of topics. But the Review Matrix is also very useful in 2 other ways in the actual writing of the synthesis. The Matrix helps you think about which topics to cover in the synthesis. The organization of the synthesis you write will not be identical to the column topics listed across the top of your Review Matrix, but those column topics may help you think about which issues to include."

Professor Dickerson pointed to Caroline's Review Matrix, continuing "The most practical way to use the Review Matrix, however, is to read down each column and think about how the studies vary or how they are alike. For example, look at the variations in number of subjects across the studies."

Caroline re-examined the Review Matrix she had prepared and began to see the variations Professor Dickerson was talking about. "I hadn't realized how much the studies differed," she commented. "At first they all looked pretty much alike. Actually, when I began doing this review of the literature, I had the sense that there was nothing left to study. It seemed like all the research questions had been asked and answered."

Professor Dickerson smiled and replied, "Yes, that's the sense that most people have when they first begin to read the scientific literature on a specific topic. By constructing a Review Matrix, however, you begin to see where the holes are. The Review Matrix helps you realize which areas appear to be missing and which topics have been covered pretty thoroughly.

But it is important," he cautioned, "if you see what you think is an area or aspect that is missing, then try to find other studies in which the missing topic has been studied. In other words, is it missing because no one has studied that aspect of the field, or is it because you didn't do a thorough enough job of finding all the studies?"

"Okay, I understand." Caroline looked at her professor and continued in a firm voice, "But this afternoon, I have to write the first draft of the synthesis for my thesis. What do I begin with? Then what do I write next? How do I organize this synthesis?"

Professor Dickerson took out a blank sheet of paper and made some notes as he talked, "Keep in mind that the organization will vary depending on your purpose. But as we discussed before, one structure you could use might be the following: describe the purpose of your literature review; summarize briefly the characteristics of the search process; describe the structure you are going to follow in writing this synthesis, in other words, the topics you are going to summarize; discuss the similarities and differences across the studies under each topic; and finally, describe your interpretation of what this means. In your interpretation, state your opinion, based on your logical and critical analysis of the literature. Include your thoughts about what is known based on this research, what hasn't been adequately covered, and what is missing. If you have some suggestions about how you would address these inadequacies, then describe them. In writing the section on your interpretation, be sure to make it clear that these are your opinions and not those of the authors of the papers."

Caroline gathered together her papers and prepared to leave. "I feel that I really know this literature," she said. "Well, I have a good sense of what this set of articles covers, anyway," she amended. "For me, the Review Matrix was most helpful in making me concentrate on the same set of topics in reading each paper."

Professor Dickerson nodded and replied, "You'll also find that the Review Matrix is very helpful in the writing process too. I'll be interested in seeing how your first draft of the synthesis turns out."

REFERENCES

1. Ueland B. *If You Want to Write.* 10th ed. St Paul, MN: Graywolf Press; 1997.
2. Rhodes R. *How to Write: Advice and Reflections.* New York: William Morrow and Company, Inc; 1996.

3. Goldberg N. *Writing Down the Bones: Freeing the Writer Within*. Boston, MA: Shambhala Publications; 1986.

4. Strunk W, White EB. *Elements of Style*. New York: Macmillan; 1979.

5. O'Conner PT. *Woe Is I: The Grammarphobe's Guide to Better English in Plain English*. East Rutherford, NJ: Putnam Publishing Group; 1996.

6. Garrard J. *Health Sciences Literature Review Made Easy: The Matrix Method*. Gaithersburg, MD: Aspen Publishers, Inc.; 1999.

Applications Using the Matrix Method

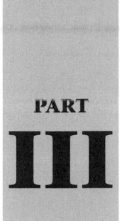

A Library of Lit Review Books

The purpose of this chapter is to describe what a Library of Lit Review Books is and why it is worth developing and maintaining. The concept is simple, but one that can buy you time and efficiency in the future. The Matrix Method provides a process for doing a review of the literature; this chapter tells you what to do afterwards. The four sections of this chapter are as follows:

☑ What Is a Library of Lit Review Books?
☑ How To Create a Library of Lit Review Books
☑ How To Use a Library of Lit Review Books
☑ Caroline's Quest: Building a Library of Lit Review Books

WHAT IS A LIBRARY OF LIT REVIEW BOOKS?

A Library of Lit Review Books is a collection of 3-ring binders, 1 for each literature review. Think of a shelf in your home or office laden with Lit Review Books—that is your library. Even 1 Lit Review Book makes a library. Just storing Lit Review Books, however, is not sufficient. This is a resource that is useful only if 2 additional conditions are met: the Lit Review Books are updated periodically and you create and use some kind of indexing system so you know what is available.

Advantages of a Library of Lit Review Books for You

Organizing Lit Review Books into a library and keeping them up to date buys you time and efficiency in the future. This resource also has the practical advantage of saving money; you do not have to photocopy an article or source document repeatedly because now you can find the first copy you made. With an initial review of the literature, you make a one-time investment in time, effort, and money. By creating and maintaining a Library of Lit Review Books, you will benefit from the interest on that investment in the future.

HOW TO CREATE A LIBRARY OF LIT REVIEW BOOKS

A literature review usually is done in a flurry of activity, with an intense effort focused on getting the synthesis written and the product produced, whether it is a paper, a grant proposal, or a final report. Afterwards, the by-products of this effort are set aside—the photocopied articles, the notes, the Review Matrix—until they are needed again. Usually the impetus for returning to a Lit Review Book is the need for a particular source document that you know was part of the initial review.

The secret to buying yourself efficiency in the future is knowing where your Lit Review Books are and keeping them up-to-date. Knowing where they are is easy—label each of your Lit Review Books and put them all together in the same place in your office. Keeping your Lit Review Books up-to-date is another matter that takes time and self-discipline. As you come across new studies, photocopy and add each to its respective Lit Review Book. An alternative is to let new documents accumulate in a safe place, then, in a moment of compulsivity, file them in the Documents section of the appropriate Lit Review Book.

Expanding the Documents section is not the only reason for updating a Lit Review Book. Additions to the Paper Trail might include new, topical web sites or lecture notes from subsequent courses. Consider setting aside one part of the Paper Trail to store notes from scientific meetings you attended after the synthesis was written. You don't have to know exactly how you will use these added materials in the future, but you do need a dependable storage system in order to find them when you need them. A Library of updated Lit Review Books provides such a system.

HOW TO USE A LIBRARY OF LIT REVIEW BOOKS

An updated and indexed Library of Lit Review Books can be very useful as you progress through your student or professional career. One of its primary uses is as a catalog over time. Simply finding things is a fundamental problem; trying to find things you know you have but can't lay your hands on is a fundamentally frustrating problem. A Library of Lit Review Books provides a permanent storage system that you can use from course to course and year to year.

A second use is that of integrating information across topics or content areas. Whether you are a graduate student, researcher, policy analyst, or writer, inevitably, you will find yourself doing more than 1 review of the literature. Even when your literature review is on a single topic, you may find it necessary to delve into several different subjects, possibly with a review and synthesis of each. For example, if you are conducting research on the effects of penicillin as a treatment for ear infections in children you might need to review the literature on the clinical effectiveness of penicillin and later conduct a separate review on ear infections and still later do a third review of papers on research methodologies used to study patient outcomes of clinical treatment. For each of these topics you could create a separate Lit Review Book, especially if the review has a complex Paper Trail or a large number of source documents in the Documents section. Your review of studies on the treatment of ear infections then might result in 3 Lit Review Books: 1 labeled Penicillin Treatment; a second, Ear Infections; and a third, Research Methods.

Following completion of the synthesis on penicillin treatment, you might use the Lit Review Book on Research Methods as your central file for methodological papers and notes. Thus, the Lit Review Book created for one review could be useful in a multitude of other reviews.

A Library of Lit Review Books that has been kept up-to-date can be a valuable resource for a group of people, such as a research team or collaborators on a project. A Library can serve as a central archive, making it easier for team members to store and find commonly used materials. This also has the advantage of increasing the opportunity for shared knowledge. Let the rules for keeping the Library up to date be simple: anyone can add an article or source document to the appropriate Lit Review Book in the Library, but the same person also has to take the responsibility of notifying other team members about the new addition by posting the addition in an indexing system on a server or updating the printed list at the beginning of the Documents section. A central archive buys time and effort for the team and reduces the photocopying bill because multiple copies of the same article do not have to be made and stored in each individual's Lit Review Book.

Caroline's Quest: Building a Library of Lit Review Books

In addition to working on her master's thesis, Caroline also had several term papers to write in some of her other courses. In her developmental psychology course, Caroline reviewed the literature on differences in self-esteem between male and fe male adolescents. Some of the research articles she included in that review were the same papers she had included in her thesis.

Caroline wanted to create a reprint file that she could maintain during and after her graduate school program. Professor Dickerson suggested that she set up a reprint filing system around a library of Lit Review Books. She began with several 3-ring binders, 1 for each Lit Review Book, and filed only 1 copy of an article in a single Lit Review Book. For example, when Caroline first read an article on gender differences in self-esteem and smoking behavior, she included the study in the Lit Review Book she labeled Gender Differences. The label she used for the Lit Review Book for her thesis was Smoking — Adolescent Girls.

Caroline used the self-esteem and smoking article both in the paper she wrote for the course on adolescent development and in her thesis. The paper was filed only once, however, in the Gender Differences Lit Review Book because it was created before she began reviewing the literature for her thesis. By using the Matrix Indexing System, described in the next chapter, Caroline was able to keep track of whether or not she had a copy of an article and where each was filed.

Over the 2 years of her graduate program, Caroline accumulated 6 Lit Review Books, including 1 on Research Methods and another on Public Health Interventions. Depending on which subject the Lit Review Book covered, she included notes from national meetings and government reports. Some of these additions were included after the literature review was completed. This was her library of Lit Review Books, and her library grew over the years as she added new articles and documents during her work. An important part of maintaining that library was keeping an up-to-date record of the materials she had and where they were stored. Thus, an integral part of creating and using a Library of Lit Review Books is its integration with the Matrix Indexing System, described in the next chapter.

The Matrix Indexing System

The Matrix Indexing System, described in this chapter, consists of merging information from 3 different sources: electronic bibliographic databases, reference management software, and the Documents section of 1 or more Lit Review Books. The topics covered in this chapter are as follows:

- ☑ What Is the Matrix Indexing System?
- ☑ How To Set up a Matrix Indexing System
- ☑ How To Expand the Documents Section
- ☑ How To Efficiently Update a Literature Review
- ☑ Caroline's Quest: Using the Matrix Indexing System

WHAT IS THE MATRIX INDEXING SYSTEM?

How do you create a system for organizing materials across multiple reviews of the literature, over time as you add new source documents, and among colleagues or associates? The Matrix Indexing System was developed for just these purposes; it is a plan for organizing your references and reprints and managing this information on an ongoing basis. This indexing system can be useful throughout a professional career whether you begin using it as a student or later in your career.

The Matrix Indexing System consists of these activities:

- Merging information from 3 sources: (1) an electronic bibliographic database, such as MEDLINE, (2) reference management software, such as EndNote or ProCite, and (3) the Documents section of your Lit Review Book
- Expanding the Documents section of your Lit Review Book
- Updating a review of the literature

Advantages of a Matrix Indexing System

If you set up your initial review of the literature using the Matrix Method, then you already have a start on the Matrix Indexing System. The indexing system differs from the Matrix Method. The Matrix Method is a strategy for acquiring, analyzing, and writing a synthesis of a review of the scientific literature. In contrast, the Matrix Indexing System provides a way of coping with the myriad of things that you use or create as a result of a review of the literature. In other words, the Matrix Indexing System gives you a way to create a manageable system in the afterlife of each review of the literature. Here is how to create and use the Matrix Indexing System.

HOW TO SET UP A MATRIX INDEXING SYSTEM

You need 4 tools in order to create a Matrix Indexing System: electronic bibliographic databases, reference management software, reprints in the document section, and location labels.

Electronic Bibliographic Databases

From your own computer (or someone else's), you must be able to access 1 or more of the electronic bibliographic databases, such as MEDLINE or Current Contents, or any of those listed in Exhibit 3-3 in Chapter 3. A dozen or more electronic bibliographic databases are available to health sciences professionals, and more are being created at a rapid rate. MEDLINE is the oldest and largest of these databases in the health sciences. Check with the reference librarian at a biomedical library about new databases that have come on-line in recent months. There is also an effort under way by the National Science Foundation to encourage the development and use of electronic libraries. Their availability over the coming years might offer additional resources to professionals in the health sciences. Check out further information on the National Library of Medicine at http://www.index.nlm.nih.gov/databases/freemedl.html/.

In describing the role of an electronic bibliographic database in the Matrix Indexing System, MEDLINE is used as the example, although this indexing system applies to any of the databases described in Chapter 3 and probably to those that have not yet become available.

Reference Management Software

On your own computer, you need one of the reference management software packages, such as EndNote or ProCite. These software packages allow users to download information from an electronic bibliographic database to files on their own computers. Software packages designed to format references in research papers and reports have been available for approximately 15 years, and those on the market can be used with a variety of computer platforms, such as Macintosh, IBM, and Unix-based systems. Currently, the 2 most commonly used programs, EndNote and ProCite, have the capability of downloading information from electronic databases such as MEDLINE into reference libraries on the user's own computer.

Further information about these software packages can be found on the Internet at http://www.niles.com/ (EndNote) and http://www.risinc.com/ (ProCite).

Organizing and Printing References. You can organize references to scientific papers, books, and other source documents cited in scientific or other academic publications and arrange them in the references section of a scientific paper according to your choice of bibliographic style—this is the reference management part of these software packages. The software packages offer numerous bibliographic styles to choose from, including American Psychological Association, the Vancouver style used by many medical journals, Modern Language Association of America, *Nature, Proceedings of the National Academy of Science,* and the Turabian Reference List style based on the book, *A Manual for Writers.*[1]

In preparing a manuscript to be submitted to a journal or for a report or thesis, there is an enormous savings in time and effort in being able to switch from one bibliographic style, such as the one for the *Journal of the American Medical Association,* to that required by the *American Psychologist.* This capability alone is reason enough to put a reference management software package on your computer. Over time, however, these packages have developed additional features that are now put to use in the Matrix Indexing System.

Downloading References and Abstracts. Reference management software packages provide a link between the electronic bibliographic databases, located elsewhere such as in a biomedical library or on the Internet, to a reference library on your own computer. With this software, you can download references, including abstracts of journal articles, directly from the electronic databases such as MEDLINE to your computer, which means you do not have to retype the information on your own computer—the software does it for you. If you have difficulty downloading references and abstracts from your library, check with a reference librarian about the possibility of special instructions. Often, university based libraries conduct tutorials about how to use reference management software packages; check to see if such classes are available at your library.

Your Reference Library. You can create and maintain one or more user-specified reference libraries on your computer—the software sets these libraries up for you. Read the manual included with the software package.

You can sort references in your reference library by author, year of publication, journal, topic, or by any other category you specify. Most reference management programs also have a search capability that enables you to find articles within the references you have stored using whatever terms you choose. For example, you can find all of the articles in your own ProCite library that mention the words, "randomized clinical trial."

There is also flexibility about where you will search in your reference library. For example, you can direct the search to include the document title, the abstract, and notes you have written about the article. This is a real advantage since the likelihood of finding a source document will be increased if you include a search of the abstract. This search feature is a good reason for always downloading an abstract from the electronic bibliographic database rather than restricting yourself to just the author's name, article title, and journal issue. The manual included in the software package explains how to do this.

In addition to searching each reference in the information downloaded from the electronic bibliographic database into your own reference library, you can also create your own key words or labels, store these labels in a particular part of the reference file, and then search on those labels. Some of the programs have set aside sections just for this purpose. For example, 3 such sections provided in EndNote are Labels, Key Words, and Notes. You have to decide which section to use consistently as a place for storing your Location Label for each article. These 2 features, storing a key word in a specific location and the search capability, are especially useful in using a standard list of Location Labels to keep track of where your source documents can be found.

Reprints in the Documents Section

You need the Documents section of a Lit Review Book from 1 or more reviews of the literature. Because organization is critical to being able to find things when you need them, think of your Lit Review Book as residing on a shelf in your office.

Location Labels for Lit Review Books

Location Labels describe where you keep your reprints or other source documents. These Location Labels provide a link between the references in your reference management software and the reprints in the Documents section in one or more Lit Review Books. In creating a standard list of Location Labels, the most efficient strategy is to make this list before you do a review of the literature or accumulate reprints in the Documents section of the Lit Review Book. This means that you will need to use the reference management software package from the beginning. For example, at the initial stage of the review of the literature as you search the electronic databases for relevant papers in research journals, you can download the references and their corresponding abstracts of interesting papers into a reference library on your computer. By the time you have completed the review of the literature, you will probably have a large set of references in your reference library, only some of which have corresponding reprints in the Documents section of your Lit Review Book.

Create a list of Location Labels by tagging each reference in your reference library that has a reprint or photocopy in the Documents section of your Lit Review Book. Use a standard label, such as: Reprint—Name of Lit Review Book. For example, suppose that you have 3 Lit Review Books: one on Antidepressants, another on Depression, and a third on Research Methods. Use a Location Label for the reprints or photocopies of journal articles in the first Lit Review Book "Reprint—Antidepressants," those in the second, "Reprint—Depression," and those in the third, "Reprint—Research Methods." By always putting these labels in a specific location in the reference file, such as the Notes section or the Label section, or whatever category is available in the computer package you use, you can search these categories for specific key words to find where you stored any reprint or photocopy you have in your Lit Review Books. An example of adding this tag to the Label section of a reference is shown in Exhibit 8-1.

Exhibit 8-1 Standard Label in an EndNote File about a Reprint in the Documents Section of a Lit Review Book on Depression

Author
  Smith, Harriet
Year
  1997
Title
  Differences between psychotherapy and tricyclic antidepressants in the treatment of depression
Journal
  Journal of Treatment
Volume
  67
Issue
  15
Pages
  1203–1208
Label
——> Reprint—Depression
Keywords
  depression, antidepressants, psychotherapy
Abstract
  This was a randomized clinical trial of psychotherapy and tricyclic antidepressants in which 100 female outpatients in a managed care organization were evaluated weekly on a pre-post basis. The study period was one year, and assessment with the . . . .
Notes
  Excellent methodological design with sufficient numbers of subjects ranging in age from 21 to 64 years. Results show that . . . .

Courtesy of Niles Software, Inc., Berkeley, California.

Location Labels for Materials Not Stored in the Documents Section

You may not have a photocopy of all of the documents that you abstract in your Review Matrix. Some documents may be in the form of books or chapters or reports available in your own library. Other source documents may be located elsewhere, such as those in a departmental library or a regional library. These materials may be too long to be photocopied, despite their usefulness in your review of the literature. For example, a chapter in a standard statistical methods book might be the key reference that describes an important analytic technique.

Location Labels can help you remember what these references are and where they are located. Keep track of these references by creating a set of labels analogous to the "Reprint—Lit Review Book" label. For example, instead of using the name of the Lit Review Book in the label, you might choose another standard set of words, such as "Reprint—Own Library," or "Reprint—Biomedical Library." Thus, a label such as "Reprint—Own Library" for the statistics book located on the shelf in your office might be the standard label you use to find the chapter with the analytic technique. The word, *Reprint*, is a useful common tag because it enables you to sort all references on that word alone and thus find the documents quickly and efficiently.

How the Elements are Linked

Location Labels, together with reference management software, are the keys to managing an overwhelming amount of detail about print or other materials that is accumulated in a literature review. You might store such a list in one of your Lit Review Books, or perhaps keep a master copy on your computer or in a printed form in another binder. If nothing else, tape a copy of your list of Location Labels to the back of your office door. The point is to create and use Location Labels as part of the Matrix Indexing System in order to manage the materials that you accumulate, use intensively, then leave and forget about, but need to access quickly at a later date.

An illustration of how the different elements of a Matrix Indexing System are linked together by the reference management software and the Location Labels is summarized in Figure 8-1. Specifically, references and abstracts of journal articles and other materials are downloaded from an electronic bibliographic database, such as MEDLINE, into your reference library on your computer using reference management software, such as ProCite. Using the same reference management software, you create a standard list of Location Labels and tag each reference in your reference library with its location. Usually, this location will be the Documents section in a Lit Review Book.

The advantage of storing all of your reprints chronologically in a Documents section of a Lit Review Book and then keeping track of the references in your reference library using Location Labels is that you will be able to find these materials when you need them. Thus, you create an organized storage and filing system for your reprints, rather than a random collection of articles that you can't access because you can't remember what is there or how to locate the materials you need.

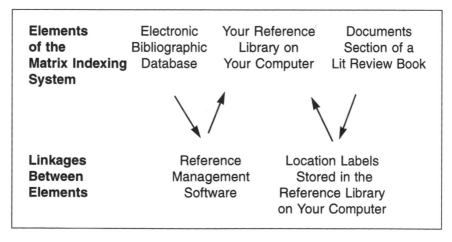

Figure 8-1 How Elements in the Matrix Indexing System Are Linked Together

HOW TO EXPAND THE DOCUMENTS SECTION

As the number of reprints you collect increases, you inevitably will be faced with the problem of running out of room in your Lit Review Book. A simple solution is to remove the Documents section from the Lit Review Book and keep the reprints in a separate 3-ring binder.

When you conduct a literature review on another topic, such as bone cancer, begin another Lit Review Book and assign a new Location Label, for example, Reprint—Bone Cancer. As the reprints in the Documents section exceed the capacity of the Lit Review Book, move them to a separate binder.

In general, using 3-ring binders to create a filing system allows you reliable and efficient access to your reprint file. A set of 3-ring binders for the reprints, used in conjunction with the other elements of the Matrix Indexing System, provides this kind of organization. Is a 3-ring binder necessary for this system to work? No, of course not. You could store all of your reprints in files, in a filing cabinet, or in boxes on a shelf. The point is, use a storage device that works for you and file your reprints logically so that you can readily retrieve them when you need them.

HOW TO EFFICIENTLY UPDATE A LITERATURE REVIEW

If you review the literature on a topic once and never look at those source documents or return to that topic again, then you can skip this section. If, however, you need to evaluate new information or consider source documents added since the original review on the same subject, then you need a strategy for updating your review of the literature. One of the simplest ways to do this is to abstract the source documents you have added since the last review and bring the Review Matrix up to date.

A typical scenario for an experienced scientist is one in which an extensive review of the literature is prepared as part of a grant proposal, then the Lit Review Book, including the

Documents section and Review Matrix, is set aside during the period when the grant is reviewed. Once the grant is awarded, then the research begins, with new references added to the Reference Library and new source documents stored in the Documents section as they become available. Later, in preparing scientific papers about the results of the study, another thorough review of the literature is needed, probably with a more specific focus than in the grant proposal. The same Lit Review Book can be used for all 3 purposes: generation of the initial literature review for the proposal, a Documents section for storing and adding reprints of source documents over time, and the preparation of the literature review for the manuscript describing the results of a completed study. Over the same period of time, from grant proposal to publication of research results, both the Reference Library and the Lit Review Book have kept pace with the researcher.

In general, updating a review of the literature is more efficient, more thorough, and quicker if the materials are organized and updated as you go along. Materials such as a Reference Library, which might be available on a server that can be accessed by all members of a research team, and the Lit Review Book, which might be stored in a central location for the same team, are invaluable resources that will help advance the research effort.

Caroline's Quest: Using the Matrix Indexing System

In her review of the literature, Caroline was interested in exploring the possibility of a link between smoking by teenage girls and depression. As an initial step, she searched for a review article on depression. The process she used illustrates the Matrix Indexing System, from identifying the paper in the electronic bibliographic database to downloading the abstract with her reference management software to making a note that she had a copy of the article in the Documents section of a Lit Review Book.

Caroline began by logging onto the OVID system through the biomedical library at her university and searched for a review article that she had identified earlier, one by Leon, Klerman, and Wickramaratne.[2] The reference in MEDLINE is shown in Figure 8-2.

She downloaded the reference and abstract, shown in Figure 8-3, onto her desktop computer. Although the appearance of the downloaded reference and abstract changed slightly between the on-line version and its downloaded version on her computer, the information was essentially the same, as shown in Figure 8-4.

Using EndNote, which was the reference management software Caroline had on her computer, she imported the reference and abstract into her reference library. The inclusion of the Leon, Klerman, and Wickramaratne reference, shown in Figure 8-5, was inserted alphabetically in Caroline's EndNote reference library, Teenagers & Smoking References.

In the standard EndNote abstract form, shown in Figure 8-6, Caroline also made a note that she had a reprint of the entire article stored in the Documents section of her Lit Review Book on Depression. This notation is shown as "Reprint—Depression" under Label in Figure 8-6.

Several days later, Caroline met with Professor Dickerson to discuss her progress. By this point she had a large file of reprints and was having trouble getting them all into her Lit Review Book. She asked, "What do you do when there are too many reprints for your binder? I can't keep buying bigger and bigger 3-ring notebooks."

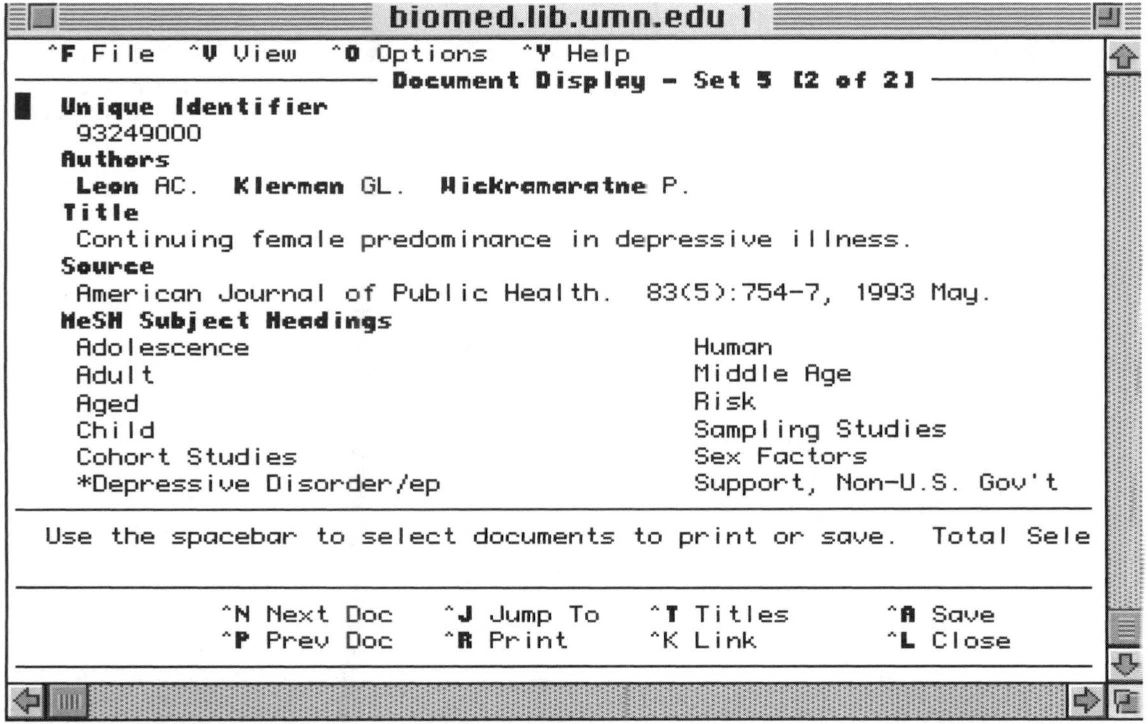

Figure 8-2 Abstract of Article in MEDLINE, Accessed by Caroline through the OVID System. *Source:* Computer screens courtesy of OVID, New York, New York. Abstract adapted with permission from A.C. Leon et al., Continuing Female Predominance in Depressive Illness, *American Journal of Public Health*, Vol. 83, No. 5, pp. 754–757, © 1993, The American Public Health Association.

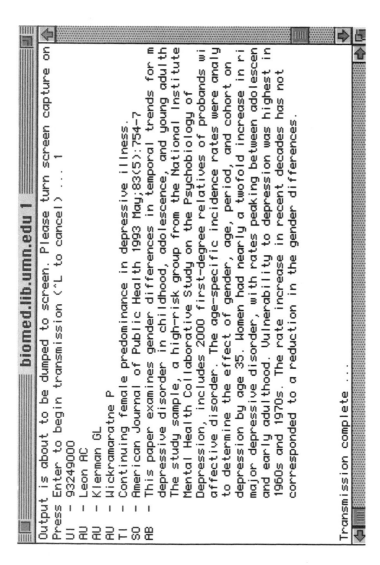

Figure 8-3 Reference and Abstract of an Article in MEDLINE That Caroline Saved. *Source:* Computer screens courtesy of OVID, New York, New York. Abstract adapted with permission from A.C. Leon et al., Continuing Female Predominance in Depressive Illness, *American Journal of Public Health*, Vol. 83, No. 5, pp. 754–757, © 1993, The American Public Health Association.

UI – 93249000
AU – Leon AC
AU – Klerman GL
AU – Wickramaratne P
TI – Continuing female predominance in depressive illness.
SO – American Journal of Public Health 1993 May;83(5):754–7
AB – This paper examines gender differences in temporal trends for major depressive disorder in childhood, adolescence, and young adulthood. The study sample, a high–risk group from the National Institute of Mental Health Collaborative Study on the Psychobiology of Depression, includes 2000 first–degree relatives of probands with affective disorder. The age–specific incidence rates were analyzed to determine the effect of gender, age, period, and cohort on depression by age 35. Women had nearly a twofold increase in risk of major depressive disorder, with rates peaking between adolescence and early adulthood. Vulnerability to depression was highest in the 1960s and 1970s. The rate increase in recent decades has not corresponded to a reduction in the gender differences.

Figure 8-4 Abstract of a MEDLINE Article after It Was Downloaded to Caroline's Computer Prior to Its Being Imported into EndNote. *Source:* Computer screens courtesy of OVID, New York, New York, and Niles Software, Inc., Berkeley, California. Abstract adapted with permission from A.C. Leon et al., Continuing Female Predominance in Depressive Illness, *American Journal of Public Health*, Vol. 83, No. 5 pp. 754–757, © 1993, The American Public Health Association.

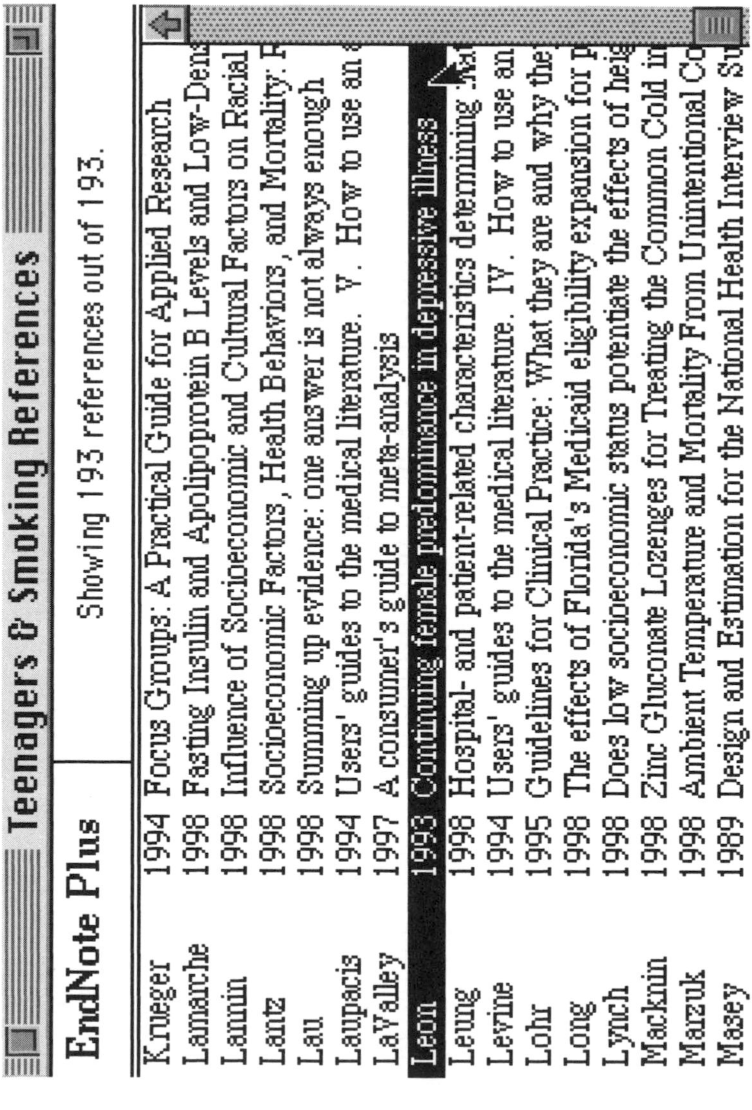

Figure 8-5 Example of an EndNote Reference Library Showing the Article That Caroline Downloaded from MEDLINE to Her Reference Library on Teenagers and Smoking References. Courtesy of Niles Software, Inc., Berkeley, California.

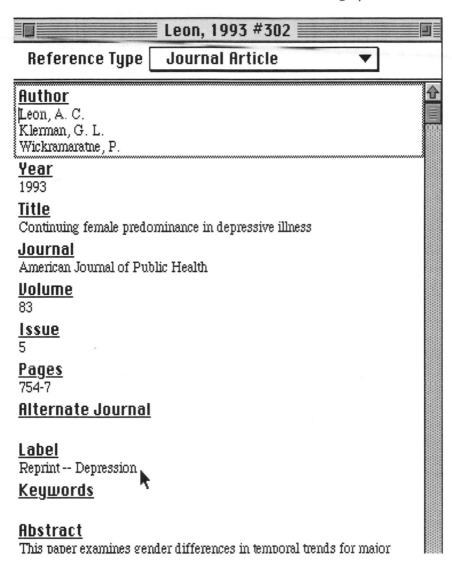

Figure 8-6 EndNote Abstract of an Article That Caroline Downloaded from MEDLINE and Her Notation of a Copy of the Article in the Documents Section of Her Lit Review Book on Depression. Courtesy of Niles Software, Inc., Berkeley, California.

"Well," he told her, *"when that happens, simply pull the Documents section out of the Lit Review Book and give it a separate binder of its own."* He pointed to a shelf in his office, continuing, *"For example, the 109 reprints I have on depression require 3 binders, which I've separated chronologically for reprints published in 1980–1989, 1990–94, and 1995–present. All are labeled Reprint—Depression in the Reference Library on my computer. Since they are indexed by year of publication, neither my students nor I have any problem finding a specific reprint."*

Caroline made a note of Professor Dickerson's strategy for handling too many reprints, and then returned to a discussion of her use of the Matrix Indexing System. *"I guess this system could be used with any kind of literature review,"* she reflected, *"whether or not it is of the scientific literature."*

Professor Dickerson described how a colleague who was an author of a series of books on gardening used the Matrix Indexing System for keeping track of his notes, gardening catalogs, and reprints from popular magazines about gardening tips. *"It really is a sensible way of organizing a lot of material,"* he agreed.

REFERENCES

1. Turabian KL. *A Manual for Writers of Term Papers, Theses and Dissertations.* 6th ed. Chicago: University of Chicago Press; 1996.
2. Leon AC, Klerman GL, Wickramaratne P. Continuing female predominance in depressive illness. *AJPH.* 1993; 83: 754–757.

Matrix Applications by Health Sciences Professionals

The purpose of this chapter is to describe examples of how the Matrix Method and the Matrix Indexing System can be used in some of the more advanced research and development activities in the health sciences. These examples are included in the following six sections in the chapter:

- ☑ What Are Matrix Applications?
- ☑ How To Use Matrix Applications in a Research Project
- ☑ How To Use Matrix Applications in a Meta-analysis
- ☑ How To Use Matrix Applications in Developing Clinical Practice Guidelines
- ☑ How To Use Matrix Applications in Evidence-Based Medicine
- ☑ Caroline's Quest: Matrix Applications in a Nonscientific Setting

WHAT ARE MATRIX APPLICATIONS?

A Matrix application is the use of the concepts and procedures of either the Matrix Method, the Matrix Indexing System, or both. The Matrix Method is a plan for gathering materials to be included in a review of the literature, systematically analyzing the information and writing a synthesis, and organizing and filing documents, notes, and other materials in 1 of 4 sections (Paper Trail, Documents section, Review Matrix, and Synthesis) in a Lit Review Book during and after completion of the review. The Matrix Indexing System is a set of procedures for bringing together and accessing information from 3 locations: (1) references obtained from electronic bibliographic databases, (2) a reference library on your computer, and (3) copies of scientific papers and other materials kept in the Documents section of your Lit Review Book.

Advantages of Matrix Applications

Used either separately or together, the Matrix Method and the Matrix Indexing System offer an efficient strategy that can be used throughout the career of a health sciences professional in a variety of settings, including

- academia;
- research and evaluation consulting firms;
- clinical settings such as a private practice or managed care organization;
- city, county, and state departments of health and public health;
- government and health policy organizations responsible for policy analysis or development of health legislation and regulations;
- research and development departments in private sector, health-related industries such as pharmaceutical or medical electronics companies;
- consumer health information organizations such as those that produce science magazines and newsletters, patient information brochures for managed care organizations or

hospitals, and health and science sections of daily newspapers.

Matrix Applications can be used by an individual or by a group or team of people. For example, in setting up a Matrix Indexing System for use by a group, the reference library created with reference management software such as ProCite could be maintained on an office computer that is accessible to all members of a research or development team. Reprints of the research papers and other scientific articles filed chronologically in the Documents section also could be maintained in a central location, and a system for adding new source documents and accessing them could be developed among members of the team.

When used in conjunction, the Matrix Method and the Matrix Indexing System offer a versatile and effective strategy for conducting a review of the literature and maintaining a library of reprints by an individual or group in a variety of settings. This is a cost- and time-efficient strategy for the busy health sciences professional. Examples of how this strategy can be used in the context of different kinds of activities are described in the remainder of this chapter.

The example used in Caroline's Quest at the end of this chapter departs from the traditional scientific setting and describes how Matrix applications can be modified and used in preparing background information for a lay audience. Whether the author's intent is to communicate research findings to a group of scientists or to describe the latest breakthrough in medicine to readers of the morning newspaper, Matrix applications can be used to organize the writer's notes and thoughts.

HOW TO USE MATRIX APPLICATIONS IN A RESEARCH PROJECT

A typical research project has several different stages of development, from the conception of the idea to publication of the final results. These stages may vary depending on the researcher, the reason for doing the project, and the goals of the research. In an academic setting, research projects in the health sciences generally follow these 3 stages: (1) preparation of a proposal describing the hypothesis and methods for carrying out the study (sometimes this is a grant proposal, which is a request for funding of the study); (2) implementation of the project once approval or funding has been obtained; and (3) preparation of the written reports and papers to be submitted for publication in peer-reviewed journals.

The Matrix Method and Matrix Indexing System can be used to access, analyze, and manage references, reprints, and reviews of the literature at each of these 3 stages in the research process. Application of these tools also can have a cumulative advantage as the information and the files acquired at each stage build on those gathered at the previous stage.

For example, preparing a grant proposal is rarely a linear activity that progresses in lockstep from the generation of an idea, to reviewing of the literature, to planning the methodology, to writing the proposal. In reality, these activities occur more or less simultaneously. Although each of these tasks may dominate the researcher's time and attention at any point in time, there is often the need to recheck the literature while in the midst of planning the methodology or to rethink the research questions as plans for the proposed analysis are being finalized.

Most experienced researchers will have a working knowledge of the research literature as they think about ideas for a new study for months or even years. As these thoughts germinate, additional possibilities for studies may be suggested in publications or presentations at scientific meetings or in discussions with colleagues. Additional publications, such as newly published journal articles, can be stored in the Documents section of a Lit Review Book and indexed in the Reference Library on the scientist's computer.

When ideas for a research study begin to take shape, a more intensive effort may be mounted to systematically review the literature, especially on topics tangentially related to the research idea or to methodological approaches that might be applicable. At this point, a Review Matrix can be set up, the choice of column topics made, and the research literature abstracted.

Finally, when the grant proposal or other research document is written, the intensity will increase in tracking down specific references or locating studies in areas in which there appear to be gaps in the knowledge base. This is the point when a synthesis is written, based on the literature abstracted in the Review Matrix.

By developing and maintaining a Matrix Indexing System from the "mulling-over" period to its use in the preparation of a Review Matrix, researchers can accumulate the materials they need to abstract the literature and write a concise synthesis. Often there is a strict limitation on the number of pages in a grant proposal. The literature review, which is one small part of the proposal, has to be accurate, thorough, and concise. For example, most NIH grant proposals have a 25-page limit, of which the literature review is a very small part. Therefore, previous knowledge about the topic has to be distilled and thoroughly accurate. The Review Matrix is a useful tool in this distillation process.

Once the research project is funded, the researcher will continue to read the scientific literature and add new publications to the Reference Library, using reference management software such as EndNote or ProCite to maintain an up-to-date reprint file of the relevant studies. Later, when the project has progressed to the preparation of scientific papers or reports, the health scientist with an up-to-date Documents section in the Lit Review Book and an equally current Reference Library on his or her own computer is in a good position to update the Review Matrix of previously abstracted papers and write a synthesis for the papers.

HOW TO USE MATRIX APPLICATIONS IN A META-ANALYSIS

A meta-analysis consists of the statistical evaluation of multiple research studies or clinical trials on a specific topic. Standardized procedures for conducting a meta-analysis are summarized in Chapter 3, and some historical background about the development of the meta-analytic technique is described in Chapter 1.

The procedures for a meta-analysis require that a study protocol be clearly specified. The first task is to describe the purpose, the methodology, and especially the criteria for selecting studies. Next, the studies to be analyzed must be selected and reviewed. Finally, the statistical procedures for summarizing the results are applied to the set of studies included in the analysis.

The Matrix Method provides a structure for carrying out the first 2 stages of a meta-analysis. For example, the criteria for the kinds of studies to be gathered and a complete record of how the literature was searched can be documented in the Paper Trail section of the Lit Review Book. Once the studies for the meta-analysis are selected, they can be assembled and filed chronologically in the Documents section. Then the critical elements of purpose and research methodology can be abstracted in a Review Matrix. The information needed for the statistical analysis can also be included as column topics in the Review Matrix.

The advantage of using the Matrix Method becomes even more apparent if the meta-analysis is being done by 2 or more people. Often, a large number of scientific papers have to be reviewed before a final decision is made about which studies meet the criteria. This task could be assigned to 2 or more people who use a Review Matrix with the same set of column topics. Then the final selection of the studies to be included in the meta-analysis could be based on the information abstracted in their Review Matrices.

The primary emphasis in a meta-analysis is on the statistical summary of empirical studies and the interpretation of those results; however, these end points could be compromised by the ways in which the tasks of selecting and reviewing the basic materials—the studies to be analyzed—are carried out. The Matrix Method and the Matrix Indexing System provide an additional level of organization and efficiency in rigorously accomplishing those fundamental tasks for a meta-analysis.

While this guide is tailored largely to graduate students for use in an academic setting, the Matrix Method and the Matrix Indexing System are applicable to research in other arenas as well. The following 2 sections outline the use of the Matrix applications for developing clinical practice guidelines and for performing research for evidence-based medicine.

HOW TO USE MATRIX APPLICATIONS IN DEVELOPING CLINICAL PRACTICE GUIDELINES

Practice guidelines give health care providers such as physicians, nurses, and allied health professionals sound strategies for delivering the best possible health care based on the scientific literature. Although practice guidelines initially were created by nationally based teams of health care professionals under the sponsorship of organizations such as the Agency for Health Care Research and Policy, recently, such development has shifted to more local or regional groups made up of clinicians within managed care organizations, health care reimbursement companies, and even small practice groups.

The fundamental concept in developing a clinical practice guideline is to create a set of best practices for diagnosing, treating, managing, or preventing a clinical condition based on the scientific literature. Regardless of what practice guideline is being developed, a review of the literature is a necessary step, and Matrix applications can be an integral part of this phase of the development of a practice guideline.

Consider, for example, a team of clinicians in an outpatient clinic consisting of a pediatric nurse-practitioner, pediatrician, and telephone triage or intake nurse who work together to develop a practice guideline on otitis media (middle ear infection) in young children. After agreeing on the definition of the condition and the criteria for the guideline, they divide up the task of reviewing the literature based on the process and the structure of the Matrix Method.

The intake nurse reviews the literature on symptoms of the condition; the pediatrician focuses on current research on treatment and clinical management; and the nurse-practitioner concentrates on studies about prevention of otitis media at the individual and community levels. By coordinating their efforts through the use of a single Lit Review Book, the task is accomplished in less time than it would take an individual. For example, they meet to agree on the criteria for the search, maintain a log of the strategies they used and the electronic databases and other sources they consulted, and generate an ongoing list of key words. This information is recorded in the Paper Trail section of their Lit Review Book, which is stored in a central location. The documents they gather, including reprints of studies, examples of guidelines from other groups, and papers from secondary and tertiary sources such as the Cochrane Library, are filed in the Documents section. Later in the process, they make a joint decision about the column topics to be included in a Review Matrix.

In abstracting the documents in the Review Matrix, the strategy they choose is to have all 3 team members carefully read all of the documents, but have different members abstract a subset of the column topics. For example, the nurse-practitioner abstracts all of the documents for column topics concerned with treatment and management, and the pediatrician abstracts the same set of articles on recognition of symptoms. Thus, by the time the guideline is ready to be written, all of the team members are thoroughly versed in the scientific literature.

In this example, the column topics might include methodological issues, but the main focus is on the major subheadings of the guideline, such as symptom recognition, diagnosis, treatment, management, and prevention. The purpose of the guideline will dictate the choice of column topics for the Review Matrix.

The Matrix Indexing System would also be an asset in preparing a clinical guideline as the literature is being reviewed and then later in updating the guideline. For example, once a year, a member of the original team of developers uses the same search strategy with the same electronic bibliographic database, such as MEDLINE, to identify new studies on the same topic. During the same period of time, team members or any of the other practitioners in the outpatient clinic, add scientific papers or other materials to the Documents section of the Otitis Media Lit Review Book and update the reference library, which is on a centrally located office computer. One person in the clinic is designated as the individual responsible for coordinating all Lit Review Books on a variety of clinical topics of interest to the clinicians.

In summary, Matrix applications will not accomplish all of the tasks needed to develop clinical practice guidelines, but they can provide an efficient process and a well-defined structure for accomplishing the task. Matrix applications can also be especially useful when a team of health professionals must coordinate their efforts to produce a single product in the form of a guideline for the care of patients with a specific condition.

HOW TO USE MATRIX APPLICATIONS IN EVIDENCE-BASED MEDICINE

Evidence-based medicine is as much a philosophy about the importance of using current research findings as a basis for clinical decisions as it is a series of well-defined Users' Guides for understanding how to read and interpret the literature. Currently, there are 20 Users' Guides and more are expected in the future.[1-20] The Matrix Method and Matrix Indexing System are consistent with the principles of evidence-based medicine and can provide a structure and process for implementing this approach.

Consider, for example, a nurse-practitioner in a diabetes clinic who wants to develop an outpatient program on diet and exercise for her elderly patients that would emphasize improvement in their quality of life. She begins by reading the Users' Guide published in the 1997 issue of *JAMA* on how to use articles about health-related quality of life.[17] Once she understands the principles of this type of research as described in that Users' Guide, she begins her search of the current literature. She also stores a copy of the Users' Guide in front of the Paper Trail section of her Diabetes Lit Review Book in order to have it handy.

Using the principles of the Matrix Method, she looks up the Users' Guide on MEDLINE and records the MeSH headings, some of which include quality of life, quality-adjusted life years, and patient care planning. She then searches MEDLINE for this type of article in combination with key words describing the condition such as diabetes, diet, and exercise. She also examines the list of references at the end of the Users' Guide on health-related quality of life in order to identify studies that might be related to her topic of interest.

Although her focus is on the quality of life of elderly people, she realizes that research in this area is relatively recent and might not have included people over 65 years of age. For that reason, she does not limit her MEDLINE search by age of subjects. She keeps notes in the Paper Trail section of her Lit Review Book on the key words, procedures, and search strategies she used.

After reviewing references and abstracts of the studies online, she downloads the references from MEDLINE into a reference library on her computer using EndNote. Next she goes to the biomedical library, examines specific articles, and photocopies those that are most relevant to her topic. These she files in the Documents section of her Lit Review Book.

In deciding which column topics to use in setting up the Review Matrix, the nurse-practitioner again consulted the Users' Guide on health-related quality of life. She included as column topics some of the issues raised in that article, such as whether or not the research studies she reviewed measured aspects of patients' lives that the patients themselves considered important, and characteristics of the data collection instruments, especially the validity of the questionnaire. In general, the Users' Guide helped the nurse-practitioner think about the kinds of issues she needed to consider in her own review of the literature.

After abstracting the research studies in the Review Matrix, the nurse-practitioner wrote a brief synthesis of the literature as a basis for deciding which instrument to use in measuring health-related quality of life in her clinical practice. In the process of identifying research studies from MEDLINE, she created a reference library on health-related quality of life and used a Location Label to note which references had a photocopy of the complete study in the Documents section of her Quality of Life Lit Review Book.

Caroline's Quest: Matrix Applications in a Nonscientific Setting

One of the requirements of the master's degree program Caroline was enrolled in was a 3-month internship in the community. Caroline was interested in applying what she had learned in her public health courses to helping people in the community understand and use current research findings to improve their own health. She therefore chose to do her internship with a science writer for a local city newspaper. Caroline's first assignment was to do background research for a 3-part series of articles to be published in the newspaper on how to prevent injuries to children in day care centers.

The newspaper's health reporter responsible for the final writing of the series of articles was Caroline's mentor for the internship. Together, they developed an outline that Caroline would follow to gather information needed for writing the articles. The topics for the 3 articles were (1) a description of the kinds of injuries to children in day care settings and what their causes are, (2) how such injuries can be prevented, and (3) a checklist of things parents should look for in deciding whether a day care center was safe.

Caroline began by searching some of the major electronic bibliographic databases, including MEDLINE from 1985 to the present, Current Contents from 1994 to the present, and CINAHL from 1982 to the present. She found 3 research studies from these sources.[21–23] She called the university's biomedical library and asked that a copy of each of the studies be faxed to her at the newspaper.

Next, Caroline called the state health department and talked to the director of the office responsible for licensing day care centers about the reporting of day care injuries. She recorded her notes on a standard interview form, shown in Exhibit 9-1. Caroline also obtained a fax copy of the statistics for fatal and nonfatal injuries to day care children over the past 5 years.

Caroline's reporter-mentor looked over the information Caroline had collected and advised her to do some telephone interviews with experts in the field.

Exhibit 9-1 Caroline's Interview Form

```
Date _____    Time _____

Person Interviewed _____
Telephone _____    ___    FAX _____
e-mail _____
Company/Organization _____
Interview Topic _____
Notes and Quotes _____
_____
_____
Additional contacts or leads suggested _____
_____
```

"How do I locate the experts?" Caroline asked. "Maybe I could try to call the authors of the research articles?" she looked inquisitively at the reporter.

Her mentor smiled, "Yes, but a quicker way to solve that problem would be to contact the people at ProfNet and find out if there are any local experts with information that would be of interest to the readership of this newspaper."

"What's ProfNet?" Caroline asked.

"It's an Internet service staffed by public relations experts at colleges and universities across the country that provides journalists and authors with leads on expert sources from more than 2,000 colleges, universities, think tanks, national laboratories, hospitals, nonprofit organizations, corporations, and public relations agencies. It was founded in 1993. Look up their web site at http://www. profnet.com/whatisprofnet.html/. The ProfNet section you should access for this series of articles is Healthcare/Medicine/Pharmaceuticals/Biotechnology."

As a result of her inquiries of ProfNet, Caroline contacted professors at 2 nearby universities and a staff person at a nonprofit organization for prevention of childhood injuries. She recorded her notes from each interview on her standardized interview form.

During the first week of her internship, Caroline also searched other sites on the Internet, such as some of the leading newspapers, state and federal agencies responsible for regulation of day care centers, and local and statewide associations of licensed day care providers. From these sources, she identified parents, day care providers, and community leaders who were willing to be interviewed. She called several people from each of these categories.

Caroline used the Matrix Method to organize the information she collected for the newspaper assignment. First, she created a Lit Review Book with the standard 4 sections: Paper Trail, Documents Section, Review Matrix, and Synthesis. In the Paper Trail section, she documented her search activities and added a subsection on interviews where she kept a list of interviewees by date and other people they suggested that she contact. This list was actually a record of her use of the snowball technique applied to people, rather than references, as Professor Dickerson had taught her initially.

Caroline modified the standard approach of the Matrix Method to her needs in this non-scientific setting. First, she expanded the Documents section of the Lit Review Book by subdividing it into 3 sections: Research Studies, Interviews, and Statistics. Once she had collected sufficient information, Caroline broadened the idea of column topics for the Review Matrix. She used the broad headings of the 3-part series to develop 3 subtopics, consisting of research studies, interviews (further subdivided by parents, day care providers, regulators, experts, and other), and statistics. In constructing the Review Matrix, Caroline treated each type of information as a document, whether it was a research study, a set of notes on a standardized interview form, or a list of statistics. By using the Review Matrix in this way, she was better able to see what was missing and where she needed additional information. Caroline then wrote a brief, 3-page memo synthesizing the information from the Review Matrix—1 page for each of the 3 intended articles.

While in the process of preparing the Lit Review Book on Day Care Injuries, Caroline also used the Matrix Indexing System to either download information from an electronic source, such as MEDLINE, or enter notes directly into an End-Note file on her desktop computer. In addition to the standard EndNote templates for a journal article, book, or report, Caroline also had the option of using a template for a newspaper article, a personal communication (which she used to record each of the interviews), and a generic format which she used to make a record of her statistical reports.

As they were going over the final materials in preparation for writing the 3-part series, Caroline's reporter-mentor was surprised by the effort Caroline had gone to in organizing the background information. "This is a lot of work!" her mentor commented. "Usually I just keep a few notes on a yellow legal pad from which I write the article."

"I know it seems like extra effort," Caroline replied, "but actually, it's a lot easier to have it all in the same spot—in the Lit Review Book—where I can just grab the whole set when I need it. Storing everything in a Lit Review Book, together with an electronic copy of the reference library from EndNote, also helps me remember where things are for other writing assignments. I can't always remember where I put a reprint of a study or the notes of an interview, but I can usually recall which assignment I was working on. Then all I have to do is pull the Lit Review Book on that assignment."

Caroline's mentor commented, "Seems to me that the Matrix System is useful in a lot of ways when it is necessary to summarize information. I think I'll try it myself."

"Oh, yes," Caroline said a bit smugly, "it's a very useful strategy. Even from the beginning, I knew that the Matrix Method was more than just a simple spreadsheet that's called a Review Matrix."

Caroline raised her eyebrows a bit like Professor Dickerson did when he began a lecture, "The Matrix Method is a system for how to access, integrate, and use information from a variety of sources in order to prepare a written synthesis of the scientific literature. I recommend it highly."

REFERENCES

1. Guyatt GH, Rennie D. Users' Guides to the Medical Literature. *JAMA.* 1993;270:2096–2097.
2. Oxman AD, Sackett DL, Guyatt GH. Users' guides to the Medical literature: I. How to get started. *JAMA.* 1993;270:2093–2095.
3. Guyatt GH, Sackett DL, Cook DJ, Evidence-Based Medicine Working Group. Users' guides to the medical literature. II. How to use an article about therapy or prevention. A. Are the results of the study valid? *JAMA.* 1993;270:2598–2601.
4. Guyatt GH, Sackett DL, Cook DJ, Evidence-Based Medicine Working Group. Users' guides to the medical literature. II. How to use an article about therapy or prevention. B. What were the results and will they help me in caring for my patients? *JAMA.* 1994;271:59–63.
5. Jaeschke R, Guyatt G, Sackett DL, Evidence-Based Medicine Working Group. Users' guides to the medical literature. III. How to use an article about a diagnostic test. A. Are the results of the study valid? *JAMA.* 1994;271:389–391.
6. Jaeschke R, Guyatt GH, Sackett DL, Evidence-Based Medicine Working Group. Users' guides to the medical literature. III. How to use an article about a diagnostic test. B. What are the results and will they help me in caring for my patients? *JAMA.* 1994;271:703–707.
7. Levine M, Walter S, Lee H, et al. Users' guides to the medical literature. IV. How to use an article about harm. *JAMA.* 1994;271:1615–1619.
8. Laupacis A, Wells G, Richardson WS, Tugwell P, Evidence-Based Medicine Working Group. Users' guides to the medical literature. V. How to use an article about prognosis. *JAMA.* 1994;272:234–237.
9. Oxman AD, Cook DJ, Guyatt GH, Evidence-Based Medicine Working Group. Users' guides to the medical literature. VI. How to use an overview. *JAMA.* 1994;272:1367–1371.
10. Richardson WS, Detsky AS, Evidence-Based Medicine Working Group. Users' guides to the medical literature. VII. How to use a clinical decision analysis. A. Are the results of the study valid? *JAMA.* 1995;273:1292–1295.
11. Richardson WS, Detsky AS, Evidence-Based Medicine Working Group. Users' guides to the medical literature. VII. How to use a clinical decision analysis. B. What are the results and will they help me in caring for my patients? *JAMA.* 1995;273:1610–1613.
12. Hayward RS, Wilson MC, Tunis SR, Bass EB, Guyatt G, Evidence-Based Medicine Working Group. Users' guides to the medical literature. VIII. How to use clinical practice guidelines. A. Are the recommendations valid? *JAMA.* 1995;274:570–574.

13. Wilson MC, Hayward RS, Tunis SR, Bass EB, Guyatt G, Evidence-Based Medicine Working Group. Users' guides to the medical literature. VIII. How to use clinical practice guidelines. B. What are the recommendations and will they help you in caring for your patients? *JAMA*. 1995;274:1630–1632.

14. Guyatt GH, Sackett DL, Sinclair JC, et al. Users' guides to the medical literature. IX. A method for grading health care recommendations. *JAMA*. 1995;274:1800–1804.

15. Naylor CD, Guyatt GH, Evidence-Based Medicine Working Group. Users' guides to the medical literature. X. How to use an article reporting variations in the outcomes of health services. *JAMA*. 1996;275:554–558.

16. Naylor CD, Guyatt GH, Evidence-Based Medicine Working Group. Users' guides to the medical literature. XI. How to use an article about a clinical utilization review. *JAMA*. 1996;275:1435–1439.

17. Guyatt GH, Naylor CD, Juniper E, et al. Users' guides to the medical literature. XII. How to use articles about health-related quality of life. *JAMA*. 1997;277:1232–1237.

18. Drummond MG, Richardson WS, O'Brien BJ, Levine M, Heyland D, Evidence-Based Medicine Working Group. Users' guides to the medical literature. XIII. How to use an article on economic analysis of clinical practice. A. Are the results of the study valid? *JAMA*. 1997;277:1552–1557.

19. O'Brien BJ, Heyland D, Richardson WS, Levine M, Drummond MF, Evidence-Based Medicine Working Group. Users' guides to the medical literature. XIII. How to use an article on economic analysis of clinical practice. B. What are the results and will they help me in caring for my patients? *JAMA*. 1997;277:1802–1806.

20. Dans AL, Dans LF, Guyatt GH, Richardson S, Evidence-Based Medicine Working Group. Users' guides to the medical literature. XIV. How to decide on the applicability of clinical trial results to your patient. *JAMA*. 1998;279:545–549.

21. Strauman-Raymond K, Lie L, Kempf-Berkseth J. Creating a safe environment for children in day care. *Journal of School Health*. 1993;63:254–257.

22. Bernardo LM. Parent-reported injury-associated behaviors and life events among injured, ill, and well preschool children. *Journal of Pediatric Nursing*. 1996;11:100–110.

23. Wiliams AF, Wells JAK, Ferguson SA. Development and evaluation of programs to increase proper child restraint use. *Journal of Safety Research*. 1997;28:197–202.

Useful Resources for Literature Reviews

PURPOSE

This appendix consists of lists of sources and resources that may be useful in searching for information as you review the literature. Resources on the Internet as well as the more standard print sources are provided. Web site addresses were accurate at the time this book went to press, but these addresses can change, and the author and publisher assume no responsibility for their continued accuracy. If the address is not accurate when you use it, then try using the key words of the organization in a general search for the correct address.

USEFUL REFERENCES AND LISTS FOR THE HEALTH SCIENCES PROFESSIONAL

Clinical Practice Guidelines

Electronic Source

National Academy of Sciences: Institute of Medicine http://www2.nas.edu/iom/

Print Sources

American Medical Association. Directory of Clinical Practice Guidelines: 1998 Annual Edition. Chicago: American Medical Association, 1997.

Green, E, Katz, J. (eds). *Clinical Practice Guidelines for the Adult Patient*. St. Louis: Mosby, 1994.

Lechtenberg, R, Schutta, HS. (eds). *Neurology Practice Guidelines*. New York: M. Dekker, 1998.

Oncology practice guidelines. *Oncology* 10 (11 Suppl), 1996.

US Department of Health and Human Services, Office of Disease Prevention and Health Promotion. *Guide to Clinical Preventive Services: Report of the U.S. Preventive Services Task Force*. 2nd ed., Baltimore: Williams & Wilkins, 1996. Also available at http://text.nlm.nih.gov

Periodicals about Clinical Practice Guidelines

Joint Commission on Accreditation of Health Care Organizations. *Abstracts of Clinical Care Guidelines*. 1989–present. Monthly abstracts of guidelines.

US Department of Health and Human Services, Agency for Health Care Policy and Research. *Clinical Practice Guidelines*. There are 19 issues. Each consists of 3 parts: (1) a detailed description of a practice guideline, (2) a summary of the content, and (3) a consumer. Also available in electronic form from HSTAT as free text.

Centers for Disease Control and Prevention. Morbidity and Mortality Weekly Report. Available as full text on HSTAT, also available at: http://www.cdc.gov/epo.mmwr/mmwr.html

Additional References about Clinical Guidelines

Cook, DJ, Greengold, NL, Ellrodt, AG, Weingarten, SR. The relations between systematic reviews and practice guidelines. *Annals of Internal Medicine.* 127(3):210–216.
Field, MJ, Lohr, KN. (eds). *Guidelines for Clinical Practice: From Development to Use.* Committee on Clinical Practice Guidelines, Division of Health Care Services, Institute of Medicine. Washington, D.C.: National Academy Press, 1992. Also available at: http://www.nap.edu/readingroom/records/0309045894.html
Lohr, KN. Guidelines for clinical practice: What they are and why they count. *Journal of Law, Medicine & Ethics.* Spring 1995; 23(1):49–56.
Saver, B.G. Whose guideline is it, anyway? (Editorial). *Archives of Family Medicine.* October 1996;5(9):532–534.

Evidence-Based Medicine: List of Users' Guides by Year of Publication

1993 Users' Guides

Guyatt GH, Rennie D. Users' Guides to the Medical Literature (Editorial). *JAMA.* 1993;270:2096–2097.
Oxman AD, Sackett DL, Guyatt GH. Users' guides to the medical literature: I. How to get started. JAMA. 1993;270:2093–2095.
Guyatt GH, Sackett DL, Cook DJ, Evidence-Based Medicine Working Group. Users' guides to the medical literature. II. How to use an article about therapy or prevention. A. Are the results of the study valid? JAMA. 1993;270:2598–2601.

1994 Users' Guides

Guyatt GH, Sackett DL, Cook DJ, Evidence-Based Medicine Working Group. Users' guides to the medical literature. II. How to use an article about therapy or prevention. B. What were the results and will they help me in caring for my patients? *JAMA.* 1994;271:59–63.

Jaeschke R, Guyatt G, Sackett DL, Evidence-Based Medicine Working Group. Users' guides to the medical literature. III. How to use an article about a diagnostic test. A. Are the results of the study valid? *JAMA*. 1994;271:389–391.

Jaeschke R, Guyatt GH, Sackett DL, Evidence-Based Medicine Working Group. Users' guides to the medical literature. III. How to use an article about a diagnostic test. B. What are the results and will they help me in caring for my patients? *JAMA*. 1994;271:703–707.

Levine M, Walter S, Lee H, et al. Users' guides to the medical literature. IV. How to use an article about harm. *JAMA*. 1994; 271:1615–1619.

Laupacis A, Wells G, Richardson WS, Tugwell P, Evidence-Based Medicine Working Group. Users' guides to the medical literature. V. How to use an article about prognosis. *JAMA*. 1994;272:234–237.

Oxman AD, Cook DJ, Guyatt GH, Evidence-Based Medicine Working Group. Users' guides to the medical literature. VI. How to use an overview. *JAMA*. 1994;272:1367-1371.

1995 Users' Guides

Richardson WS, Detsky AS, Evidence-Based Medicine Working Group. Users' guides to the medical literature. VII. How to use a clinical decision analysis. A. Are the results of the study valid? *JAMA*. 1995;273:1292–1295.

Richardson WS, Detsky AS, Evidence-Based Medicine Working Group. Users' guides to the medical literature. VII. How to use a clinical decision analysis. B. What are the results and will they help me in caring for my patients? *JAMA*. 1995;273:1610–1613.

Hayward RS, Wilson MC, Tunis SR, Bass EB, Guyatt G, Evidence-Based Medicine Working Group. Users' guides to the medical literature. VIII. How to use clinical practice guidelines. A. Are the recommendations valid? *JAMA*. 1995;274:570–574.

Wilson, MC, Hayward RS, Tunis SR, Bass EB, Guyatt G, Evidence-Based Medicine Working Group. Users' guides to the medical literature. VIII. How to use clinical practice guide-

lines. B. What are the recommendations and will they help you in caring for your patients? *JAMA* 1995;274:1630–1632.
Guyatt GH, Sackett DL, Sinclair JC, et al. Users' guides to the medical literature. IX. A method for grading health care recommendations. *JAMA.* 1995;274:1800–1804.

1996 Users' Guides

Naylor CD, Guyatt GH, Evidence-Based Medicine Working Group. Users' guides to the medical literature. X. How to use an article reporting variations in the outcomes of health services. *JAMA.* 1996;275:554–558.
Naylor CD, Guyatt GH, Evidence-Based Medicine Working Group. Users' guides to the medical literature. XI. How to use an article about a clinical utilization review. *JAMA.* 1996; 275:1435–1439.

1997 Users' Guides

Guyatt GH, Naylor CD, Juniper E, Evidence-Based Medicine Working Group. Users' guides to the medical literature. XII. How to use articles about health-related quality of life. *JAMA.* 1997;277:1232–1237.
Drummond MG, Richardson WS, O'Brien BJ, Levine M, Heyland D, Evidence-Based Medicine Working Group. Users' guides to the medical literature. XIII. How to use an article on economic analysis of clinical practice. A. Are the results of the study valid? *JAMA.* 1997;277:1552–1557.
O'Brien BJ, Heyland D, Richardson WS, Levine M, Drummond MF, Evidence-Based Medicine Working Group. Users' guides to the medical literature. XIII. How to use an article on economic analysis of clinical practice. B. What are the results and will they help me in caring for my patients? *JAMA.* 1997;277:1802–1806.

1998 Users' Guides

Dans AL, Dans LF, Guyatt GH, Richardson S, Evidence-Based Medicine Working Group. Users' guides to the medical literature: XIV. How to decide on the applicability of clinical trial results to your patient. *JAMA.* 1998;279:545–549.

Cochrane Reviews

A list of reviews is available at: http://www.hcn.net.au/ cochrane. See also: http://www.cochrane.org/.

List of Annual Reviews by Category

Reviews of scientific information are published annually by Annual Reviews, which is a nonprofit scientific publisher. Current information about reviews can be found at the following web site: http://www.annualreviews.org. Currently, there 27 Annual Reviews, in the following 3 categories:

Biological and Medical Sciences Publications

Annual Review of Biochemistry
Annual Review of Biophysics and Biomolecular Structure*
Annual Review of Cell and Developmental Biology
Annual Review of Ecology and Systematics
Annual Review of Entomology
Annual Review of Genetics
Annual Review of Immunology
Annual Review of Medicine
Annual Review of Microbiology
Annual Review of Neuroscience
Annual Review of Nutrition
Annual Review of Pharmacology and Toxicology
Annual Review of Physiology
Annual Review of Phytopathology
Annual Review of Plant Physiology and Plant Molecular Biology
Annual Review of Psychology*
Annual Review of Public Health*

Physical Sciences Publications

Annual Review of Astronomy and Astrophysics
Annual Review of Biophysics and Biomolecular Structure*
Annual Review of Earth and Planetary Sciences
Annual Review of Energy and the Environment*
Annual Review of Fluid Mechanics

Annual Review of Materials Science
Annual Review of Nuclear and Particle Science
Annual Review of Physical Chemistry

Social Sciences Publications

Annual Review of Anthropology
*Annual Review of Energy & the Environment**
Annual Review of Political Science
*Annual Review of Psychology**
*Annual Review of Public Health**
Annual Review of Sociology

USEFUL RESOURCES

Bopp, RE, Smith, LC. *Reference and Information Services: An Introduction* (2d ed.). Englewood, Colorado: Libraries, Unlimited; 1995.

Henley, JJ. *Writing a General Research Paper.* Roane State Community College On-line Writing Lab; 1996. Available at: http://www2.rscc.cc.tn.us/~jordan_jj/OWL/Research.html.

Hord, B. *The Research Center.* Houston Community College Systems Library; 1995. Available at: http://www.hccs.cc.tx.us/Library/Center.html.

Hord, B. *Steps in the Research Process.* Houston Community College Systems Library; 1995. Available at: http://www.hccs.cc.tx.us/Library/Center/Lobby/Steps.html.

Kuhlthau, C C. *Seeking Meaning: A Process Approach to Library and Information Services.* Norwood, NJ: Ablex Publishing; 1993.

Kuhlthau, C C. *Teaching the Library Research Process* (2d ed.). Metuchen, NJ: The Scarecrow Press; 1994.

Lamm, K. *10,000 Ideas for Term Papers, Projects, Reports & Speeches.* New York: Macmillan; 1995.

Solock, J. *Searching the Internet Part I: Some Basic Considerations and Automated Search Indexes,* [InterNIC News Web site]. Sep-

*Some of the series belong to more than 1 category.

tember 1996. Available at: http://rs.internic.net/nicsupport/nicnews/archive/september96/enduser.html.

Solock, J. *Searching the Internet Part II: Subject Catalogs, Annotated Directories, and Subject Guides* [InterNIC News Web site]. October 1996. Available at: http://rs.internic.net/nic-support/nicnews/oct96/enduser.html.

USEFUL WEB SITES OF SCIENTIFIC ORGANIZATIONS, DIRECTORIES, PRINTED JOURNALS, AND ON-LINE JOURNALS

American Anthropological Association: http://www.ameranthassn.org/. Home page of the American Anthropological Association.

American Association for the Advancement of Science: http://www.aaas.org. Home page of The American Association for the Advancement of Science (AAAS). Includes links and information to many science fields.

American Chemical Society: http://www.acs.org/. Home page of The American Chemical Society with a membership of more than 151,000 chemists and chemical engineers.

American Institute of Biological Sciences: http://www2.aibs.org/aibs/. Home page of the American Institute of Biological Sciences, with links to *BioScience Magazine.*

American Journal of Clinical Nutrition: http://www.faseb.org/ajcn/. Home page of *The American Journal of Clinical Nutrition,* which is a peer-reviewed journal that publishes basic and clinical studies relevant to human nutrition.

American Psychological Society: http://psych.hanover.edu/APS/. Home page of the American Psychological Society.

American Society for Biochemistry and Molecular Biology: http://www.faseb.org/asbmb/. Home page of the American Society for Biochemistry and Molecular Biology.

American Society of Human Genetics: http://www.faseb.org/genetics/ashg/ashgmenu.htm. Home page of the American Society of Human Genetics.

American Sociological Association: http://www.asanet.org/. Home page of the American Sociological Association.

Biologists' Control Panel: http://gc.bcm.tmc.edu:8088/bio/. Site provides many useful links for biologists, including biological databases, search tools, and information.

CAB INTERNATIONAL: http://www.cabi.org/. Emphasis on agriculture, forestry, human health and the management of natural resources, with particular attention to the needs of developing countries.

Directory of Printed Periodicals: http://www.publist.com. A free on-line service that gives access to more than 150,000 printed periodicals throughout the world. Also provided is information about how to contact publishers, obtain rights and permissions, and receive documents. Initiated on the Web in June 1998.

Enter the Spleen: http://jaka.ece.uiuc.edu/spleen. Home page of the Splenic Research Institute with information about the spleen, its history, functions, and impact on everyday life.

Federation of American Societies for Experimental Biology: http://www.faseb.org/. Home page of the Federation of American Societies for Experimental Biology.

GenBank submissions: http://www3.ncbi.nlm.nih.gov/BankIt/. Site for submitting genetic sequences and information on protein coding regions, mRNA features, and structural RNA features to the GenBank library.

Health and Behavior Alliance: hhtp://www.cfah.org/. Founded in 1997, the Alliance consists of 25 professional research societies representing over 250,000 researchers. Their purpose is to increase the priority of resources devoted to health and behavior research. Their mission and member organizations are described on their home page. The Alliance is organized by the Center for the Advancement of Health, a nonprofit policy organization that promotes an understanding of health. Funded by the John D. and Catherine T. MacArthur Foundation and Nathan Cummings Foundation, the Center offers a free newsletter that you can subscribe to by sending an e-mail to <newsletter@cfah.org>. The subject line in your e-mail should say either "subscribe" or "unsubscribe" (no quotes). See their website for back copies of the newsletter.

International Sociological Association: http://www.ucm.es/OTROS/isa/. Home page of the International Sociological Association.

Institute for Scientific Information: http//www.isinet.com/. Publisher of Current Contents® and the Science Citation Index.®

(The) Johns Hopkins University BioInformatics Web: http://www.gdb.org/. This site provides many links to biological databases and other sites of biological interest.

(The) Journal of Biological Chemistry: http://www.jbc.org/. On-line version of *The Journal of Biological Chemistry.*

(The) Journal of Cell Biology: http://www.jcb.org/. On-line version of *The Journal of Cell Biology.*

(The) Journal of Clinical Investigation: http://www.jci.org/. On-line version of *The Journal of Clinical Investigation.*

(The) Journal of Experimental Medicine: http://www.jem.org/. On-line version of *The Journal of Experimental Medicine.*

Journal of Molecular Biology: http://www.hbuk.co.uk/jmb/. Home page of the *Journal of Molecular Biology.*

Journal of Nutrition: http://nutrition.org. Published by the American Society for Nutritional Sciences. On-line version of the *Journal of Nutrition,* which publishes papers based on original research in humans and other animal species.

Journal Watch: http://www.jwatch.org/. Journal Watch began in 1987 in both an on-line and newsletter format, reviewing the general medical literature for busy clinicians.

Lymphocyte Homing Images: http://www.geocities.com/CapeCanaveral/Hangar/1962. The site shows images from lymphocyte homing research.

National Academy of Sciences: http://www.nas.edu/. Home page of the National Academy of Sciences.

National Center for Biotechnology Information: http://ncbi.nlm.nih.gov/medline/query_form.html. A searchable molecular biology subset of MEDLINE with more than 700,000 citations.

Science Magazine: http://www.sciencemag.org/. Home page of Science Magazine Online with full-text of print edition and science news section.

Science's Next Wave: http://www.nextwave.org/. A site for helping new scientists find jobs and keep up with new developments in their careers.

SciWeb—The Life Science Home Page: http://www.sciweb. com/. Provides Internet-based information and communication services addressing the needs of professionals working in the fields of biotechnology, pharmaceuticals, medical diagnostics, health care and companies servicing the bio-industry.

Society for Neuroscience: http://www.sfn.org/. Dedicated to understanding the brain, spinal cord, and peripheral nervous system.

SocioSite: http://www.pscw.uva.nl/sociosite/. Site for sociologists with a European and worldwide horizon.

UniSci homepage: http://unisci.com/. UniSci is the daily science news service of the Internet, with emphasis on American university research. Updated every day, Monday through Friday, with news from all fields of science.

(The) Vaccine Page: http://vaccines.com/. This site collects, organizes, and presents news and annotated links about vaccines for parents, patients, practitioners, researchers, and students. Material is updated continuously.

The ZareLab Homepage: http://www-zarelab.stanford.edu/. Home page of Chairman of the National Academy of Sciences and Annual Reviews Inc., Prof. Richard Zare.

Index

About the Author

Judith Garrard, PhD, is an educational psychologist and professor in the Division of Health Services Research and Policy, School of Public Health, University of Minnesota. She holds joint academic appointments in the Department of Psychiatry in the Medical School and in the College of Pharmacy. Her teaching and research activities have been on a multidisciplinary basis throughout her career. For more than 20 years she has taught graduate courses in research and program evaluation methods to students throughout the health sciences. She has also been principal investigator or collaborator on numerous multidisciplinary research projects supported by grants from the National Institute on Aging, National Institute for Neurological Diseases and Stroke, Agency for Health Care Policy Research, Health Care Financing Administration, Veterans Administration, and other nationally competitive granting agencies. Her current research studies are in the areas of pharmacoepidemiology and patient outcomes of elderly populations, with an emphasis on psychoactive medication use by patients in managed care organizations and nursing homes.